P9-CTA-005

Pet Loss and Human Bereavement

JUN 13 1997

CIH 13

Pet Loss

AND

Human Bereavement

EDITED BY

WILLIAM J. KAY, HERBERT A. NIEBURG,
AUSTIN H. KUTSCHER, ROSS M. GREY,
and CAROLE E. FUDIN

WITH THE ASSISTANCE OF
LILLIAN G. KUTSCHER

THE IOWA STATE UNIVERSITY PRESS □ AMES

SF
411
.47
P48
1995

A Foundation of Thanatology Text

630 West 168th St.

New York, N.Y. 10032

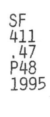

© 1984 Iowa State University Press, Ames, Iowa 50014
All rights reserved
♾ Printed on acid-free paper in the United States of America
FIRST EDITION, 1984
First paperback printing, 1988
Second paperback printing, 1995

No part of this book may be reproduced in any form or by any electronic or mechanical means, including information storage and retrieval systems, without permission in writing from the copyright holder, except for brief passages quoted in a review.

Library of Congress Cataloging-in-Publication Data
Main entry under title:

Pet loss and human bereavement.

"A Foundation of Thanatology Text."
Includes index.
1. Pet owners—Psychology. 2. Pets—Death—Psychological aspects. 3. Bereavement—Psychological aspects. I. Kay, William J.
SF411.47.P48   1984   155.9′37   83-18639
ISBN 0-8138-1326-3
ISBN 0-8138-1327-1 (paperback edition)

C O N T E N T S

FOREWORD

VETERINARIANS are beginning to recognize their opportunities and responsibilities for the emotional well-being of their clients. Companion animal veterinarians can legitimately involve themselves with the issues of emotional well-being that often directly depend upon the state of health (or disease) of their animal patients. Veterinarians and animal hospital teams are the key interfaces between pet owners and pets. The few levels of formally trained animal health workers make it incumbent upon veterinarians to be involved with the upsets of their clients. For one familiar with the profound distress experienced by pet owners faced with the death of a pet, the opportunity to reach out and create a new context for veterinary caregiving has been a personal and institutional priority.

The Animal Medical Center (New York City) is a microcosm of the far larger issue of pet-related grief and, as such, the interdisciplinary roles of its many health care workers now include the recognition of pet loss and the emotional reactions that flow from that loss. I should also not forget the effect pet loss has on other pets.

The number of people affected in a serious way by the death or dying of a pet is not known; we know pet death can be a great loss and our future studies will attempt to discover both the quantity and quality of it.

WILLIAM J. KAY, D.V.M.
Chief of Staff
Animal Medical Center
New York City

PREFACE

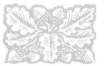

WILLIAM J. KAY
AUSTIN H. KUTSCHER

THE UNIQUE RELATIONSHIP between human pet owners and their companion animals has long been appreciated. Attesting to this phenomenon is the large group of "small animal" specialists within the veterinary medical profession — doctors of veterinary medicine practicing in urban or suburban areas where the animal patients are companion rather than utility or stock animals. For the medical director of a large urban veterinary medical center dedicated to integrated health care for animals as well as to teaching and research, daily experiences with staff, animal patients, and clients support findings recently reported by others in the human behavioral sciences. For one who has followed investigations into human reactions to separation, loss, and bereavement (the symptomatology of which has been subsumed within the medical subspecialty of thanatology), it appears that the disciplined research into human/companion animal relationships replicates information derived from anecdotal experiences related by many individuals who have endured the loss of a beloved pet. What person cannot remember an endearing quality in every pet he or she has owned? It is not difficult to document the existence of strong emotional bonding between humans and companion animals and the fact that the rupturing of such bondings can frequently result in human bereavement responses similar in quality and/or degree to those occurring when a significant person dies.

The literature abounds with clichés about the devotion and love demonstrated by pets for their owners. Behavioral scientists are discovering that these are reciprocal transactions and that for pet owners they extend beyond demonstrable emotional dimensions to a dimension that encompasses their physiological well-being. Somatization of psychic trauma becomes an actuality that must be acknowledged and attended to. This scientific adventure can be acceptable to those who have fought so long on behalf of the rights of animals and is one that engages the commitment of the veterinary medical doctor to patient and client as well as the attention of the practitioner of human medicine whose patient's bereavement is the result of the death of a pet. For both groups of health professionals, the techniques of preventive intervention on behalf of the bereaved become a major focus for caregiving.

In the past, the links between veterinary and human medicine have derived primarily from the basic and clinical sciences. Research has long been conducted (and continues to be conducted) with animals as the subjects of experimentation. Although the scientific community is frequently taken to task for the reckless abandon with which animals are sacrificed on behalf of investigations into the etiology and cure of human disease, humankind has benefited substantially from the results of this research. How many human lives have been saved because of experimental surgery first performed on animals or drugs developed after multiple trials on animal subjects? As one heroic example, we can cite the implantation of an artificial heart—the prototype of which was first implanted in a cow—into Dr. Barney Clark. As hopeless as the anticipated prognosis was in this instance, a tremendous advance in medical technology was confirmed.

Yet questions of ethical and moral significance within the parameters of human/companion animal relationships are raised in other contexts regarding the "sacrifice" of animals by some animal lovers who find a clear violation of presumed rights that are felt to almost parallel those in doctor/patient relationships. In an age so sensitive to human rights and human dignity—where it is mandated that informed consent be obtained from a patient before the initiation of medical intervention—it is not surprising to encounter pressures exerted to shield companion animals from a denial of their rights to compassionate care and a dignified death; animals employed in research are entitled to comparable concern.

Both veterinary and human medical education are challenged to introduce psychosocial aspects of caregiving into their curricula. Such programs would go beyond the physical diagnosis of pathologies and modalities of therapy, go beyond physiological anatomical structures and functions and reach into the psychosocial issues that relate to the care of the whole patient. The task in veterinary medicine involves the care of the terminally ill pet, the decisions to be made in regard to the continuation or cessation of treatment, and the relationship between the veterinarian and the pet owner during the course of the illness and after the death of the pet. Such caregiving gives sanction not only to the rights of animals to humane treatment but also to the rights of owners to find acceptance of their bereavement and respect for their emotional ties with their pets.

The contributors to this text acknowledge the significance of the human/companion animal relationship and the grief that surfaces when a pet dies or is terminally ill. As in the practice of the most enlightened caregiving for chronically or terminally ill human patients, the approach suggested involves multidisciplinary caregivers. Such a team is well represented here by veterinarians, psychiatrists, psychologists, social workers, a philosopher-ethicist, and others.

This text also deals with what has been and what may yet be learned about the human condition as derived from the human/companion animal relationship and bond—when unbroken and particularly when broken. In this crucial context and direction, future research may be especially fruitful.

Separation and loss affect human beings in diverse ways, as thanatologists have demonstrated. Through the process of grief, a bereaved survivor adjusts to separation from a loved one. When a companion animal dies, the bereavement phenomena can disrupt the normal functioning of the human survivor. The veterinarian's professional role, these authors emphasize, extends beyond that of caregiving for the pet. Veterinarians have depended on their own instinctive reactions when they offer guidance to a mourning pet owner. How much more constructive this guidance could be if supported by a more formalized knowledge base in human psychology. With the ability to offer wise and informed counsel to bereaved clients, veterinarians will expand their professional role and enhance their image as caregivers.

I

The Human/Companion Animal Bond

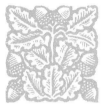

1

The Moral Status of Animals

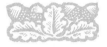

BERNARD E. ROLLIN

IN OUR SOCIETY human grief reactions to the loss of a pet animal are taken seriously as a legitimate, nonpathological phenomenon. This attitude acknowledges a fundamental intuition many people share but few can articulate: that legal and social practices notwithstanding, animals are far more than merely property.

Clearly there is a sense in which grief for a lost object can in itself be nonrational. For example, it is not rational to grieve for the loss of a car, although we may feel sorrow at our own financial misfortune. And when we grieve for the loss of an irreplaceable masterpiece in a fire, our grief is rational not because we are grieving for the work of art itself, but because it will no longer grace the lives of human beings. While it is unquestionable that this sort of consideration (awareness of *our* loss) looms large in our grief for pets, as indeed it does in our grief for departed humans, something else is operative in the case of living things.

When we grieve for living things, it is not irrational to mourn for what the dead being has lost, and thus to mourn for it in itself, as well as for ourselves and for what is missing from our lives. When a living creature — human or pet — dies, we mourn the passing of something whose life mattered to it, even if that life did not matter much to the world at large. We know that the dead person or animal can never again enjoy those activities and pleasures that were significant to its life, and for this reason we grieve.

This is why we philosophers say persons possess *intrinsic value,*

value in themselves, not merely instrumental value (use value) to others. This is why Kant says that humans must be viewed as "ends in themselves," not merely as means. And it is for this reason that we see persons as moral objects, toward whom our actions must be measured by moral categories of right and wrong, categories that simply do not fit a car or wheelbarrow.

But so, too, with pet animals. The fact that we are not thought to grieve irrationally at the death of a pet betokens the intuition that beyond our own loss, their lives mattered to them, and thus that they are of intrinsic value, that they are legitimate objects of moral concern and attention, toward whom our actions can be judged as right or wrong. It is this intuition that so desperately requires rational articulation. We all know it is easy to express our recognition of the animal's moral status and value emotionally, and even artistically. But it is much harder to give a philosophical and rational articulation of this sense of animal value which seems to be simply sloppy anthropomorphic sentimentality to many people. It is to this task we now turn, for despite its difficulty, it is of great importance to press in society for the recognition of the moral status of these animals before they die, and to try to make our social practice fit our moral intuitions.

It is interesting that historically we have ignored these intuitions about the moral status of animals. Perhaps we have repressed them because they make us too uncomfortable about our behavior toward these beings. We would expect that, at least regarding pet animals, we might have developed something of an ethic that attempts to come to grips with our relationship toward them. But despite the immense literature on ethics that exists in the West; despite the fact that philosophers have written on all sorts of things (including the claim that when we are not perceiving a chair it is not there, or that time is unreal), almost nothing has been done on the moral status of animals. We need to ask the questions: What if anything is the relevant difference between people and animals from a moral point of view? What are our moral duties to other creatures?

I shall try to present, in summary form, the results of my work in this area. I shall try to explain why there are no rational grounds for excluding animals from moral concern, and why animals have rights. Let me stress that this theory is meant as a moral ideal, which we cannot live up to instantly in our sociocultural context. But this is true of most moral ideals. Consider "turning the other cheek." Most Christians are incapable of acting that way, but the ideal is still valuable as a mark to aim at, and as a yardstick to measure conduct. Without moral theories as ideals, we tend to accept the status quo as normal, inevitable, and acceptable. Given a moral ideal, we try to make that ideal fit our sociocultural reality as far as possible. In my book, *Animal Rights and Human Morality* (1981), I develop the theory in great detail. But I also try to show how current practice regarding animals can be modified to make it much closer to this ideal. I focus specifically on research animals and pet animals, and have tried to effect real social differences in my work with veterinary students and in the federal laboratory animal bill I helped draft. Inspiring people to change the status quo is the cash value of moral philosophy.

Let us look then at the theory, and how it applies to pet animals. To begin, it is necessary to explain the concept of *morally relevant differences*. If I suddenly begin punctuating a lecture with a series of right jabs to a certain gentleman's jaw, you would ask me why I am hitting him. Suppose I said I am hitting him because he is the only person here with a red beard. That would not morally justify my hitting him. Beard color is not morally relevant here. On the other hand, if I say I saw him molesting my son before the lecture, that is morally relevant grounds for my hitting him.

The basic question, then, is: What morally relevant differences exist between people and animals? There are obviously many differences, but the question is whether they are germane to moral status or whether they are as irrelevant as beard color. Let us look very briefly at some alleged differences between humans and animals in general, before looking at pet animals in particular. These differences have all been used to claim that animals are not legitimate objects of moral attention while people are.

1. *Man has an immortal soul.* This is the classic Roman Catholic position: But is it morally relevant? (Let us ignore for a moment

our obvious inability to know who has a soul and who does not, or even what it is.) Does it justify our treating animals as less than humans? No. Cardinal Bellarmine pointed out that, if anything, it cuts the other way. Since animals do not have an immortal soul, they do not get a crack at the afterlife where wrongs are redressed. So we are actually obliged to treat them better! (Bellarmine allegedly allowed fleas to drink their fill of his blood.)

2. *Man is superior to animals (granted dominion by God; top of the evolutionary ladder).* Being superior to something does not entail its abuse. In fact, it has nothing at all to do with obligatory treatment. And anyway, how are we superior? Are we stronger? The government is stronger than any of us – does it follow that it is morally entitled to do to individuals as it sees fit? Might does not make right. Perhaps everyone drawn to this sort of argument should try the following thought experiment: Imagine a race of extraterrestrials who are smarter and superior in force to humans. Would we consider it morally justifiable for them to deny human rights, and to utilize humans for their own convenience?

From a strict evolutionary point of view, there is no top of the ladder. There is only a branching tree. If there is superiority, it has to do with species adaptability, durability, and reproductive success. In that case, the roach and the rat are right on top with humans.

Speaking in a religious context, having dominion does not mean other creatures have no rights. The Old Testament contains specific concerns about animals. And remember, parents have dominion over children – that does not mean children have no moral status.

3. *As far as domestic animals and laboratory animals are concerned, humans have regulated their lives, so these animals can be disposed of as humans see fit.* This is clearly morally irrelevant. We are causally responsible for the lives of our children, yet we cannot morally justifiably mistreat them. We do not feel that owners of slaves were morally justified in treating them as chattel, even though they, of course, had the power to do so.

4. *Animals do not feel pain.* This absurdity goes back to Descartes, who saw them as machines. If someone tells me he cannot *know* for sure that an animal feels pain, I tell him I cannot know

for sure that *he* can. I recently debated a physiologist who said that since electrochemical activity in the cerebral cortex of dogs is different from ours, dogs do not feel pain as we do. I pointed out that he does pain research on dogs and extrapolates the results to people, and rested my case. People in such organizations as the National Society for Medical Research constantly hint at the idea that animals do not feel pain, and thereby discredit themselves.

5. *Animals cannot reason or speak.* Some humans do not reason—infants, children, the senile, the insane, the comatose, the retarded—yet they are moral objects. Moreover, it is not clear that animals cannot reason. And if reason is what makes people moral objects, why do we worry about aspects of their nature that have nothing to do with reason?

Suppose we discover we can spur the rational activity of college students by wiring their seats and shocking them periodically when their attention wanders? Surely we would not consider this morally permissible. The point is that in people other factors aside from reason are morally relevant, such factors as pain and pleasure, which animals share.

6. *Social contract theory* (a version of number 4). This is the idea that morality applies only to individuals who are capable of entering into agreements with one another. For example I will respect your property on condition that you will respect mine. Only rational beings can enter into such agreements, therefore only rational beings are objects of moral concern.

Obviously this theory refers to agreements in action, mutual adjustment of behavior, rather than explicit agreements, since none of us have ever verbally agreed to a moral code. What I mean by agreement in action is exemplified by common law marriage, as recognized by the law. Although no explicit marriage contract exists, there is agreement in action, mutual adjustment, and accord in behavior.

But for a number of reasons this won't work either. Most relevant here is the fact that *pet* animals, at least, *do* stand in precisely this relationship to man, behaviorally, biologically, and evolutionarily. There is a strong social contract between humankind and dogs. The dog has given up a wild-pack nature to live in human society and function as sentinel, guardian, hunting companion, and friend in return for food, care, shelter, and pack leadership on the part of humans. We shall return to this shortly.

Let us sum up. We have seen that none of the alleged differences between humans and animals is morally relevant. In a positive vein we know also that animals possess the same features we consider morally relevant and significant in humans:
1. They are alive.
2. They have needs and interests, physical and behavioral, that matter to them — food, companionship, sex, exercise, avoidance of pain. Each animal species has a unique set of genetically programmed interests that determines its nature, or what I call, following Aristotle, its *telos*.

In human morality and in our laws we talk of our moral commitment to the needs of others in terms of their *rights* to certain treatment. When a human need or interest is central to the *nature* of a human being, we try to protect the fulfillment of that need from infringement, except in the case of the gravest social danger. So our Bill of Rights protects human rights growing out of interests we feel are central to human nature — speech, religion, assembly, property, privacy. But animals also have natures, and interests central to their natures. And if there is no morally relevant difference between humans and animals, logic leads us to conclude that animals should have rights!

The fundamental rights are obvious. First of all, the *right to life,* for without life, there is nothing to value. This means, first and foremost, we should not kill animals for trivial reasons or simply for our convenience. Equally important is the right of the animal to live in accordance with its nature. This is sometimes even more important than the right to life (as when we feel that morality forces us to euthanize an animal because it cannot live naturally, without pain). Veterinarians realize that to keep a dog "alive" when it cannot move or eat is a monstrous violation of its essential nature. Ironically this is a favor we will not afford humans, even when they ask for relief! Here, parenthetically, is an area of human morality that might be illuminated by taking animal rights seriously. We consider the person who won't euthanize a suffering dog morally culpable; why do we not feel the same way about persons or societies who will not euthanize a person who is begging to die?

In any event if animals are moral objects, we should not kill them except for morally defensible reasons, and we should not violate their natures. Furthermore we should grant their claim to our moral concern some official, socially sanctioned status in the law, which after all exists to protect moral concerns.

If we focus on the pet animal, however, we realize just how far we are from this rational ideal. As we said earlier, pet animals do have status in a social contract relationship with humans. Pet animals are vitally integrated into human society in obvious ways and in new ways, which are gradually being discovered. The dog has been part of human life for about 12,000 years — the tame wolf has been associated with human society for about 500,000 years. The dog has been shaped by society into a creature that essentially depends on us for its physical existence, satisfaction of its physical needs, behavioral needs, and social nature. Humans "created" the dog and sustain its existence. If dogs were suddenly turned loose in a world devoid of people, they would be decimated. Aside from the obvious case of chihuahas, bulldogs, and others who could simply not withstand the elements or who are too small, slow, or clumsy to be successful predators, the vast majority of all dogs would not do well. We know from the case of dogs who have gone feral that they still live on the periphery of human society, living on handouts, garbage, and vulnerable livestock, such as poultry and lambs. Without vaccination, overwhelming numbers would succumb to disease.

We, in turn, rely on the dog to be a guardian of home and family, a warrior and messenger, a sentry, a playmate for and protector of children, a guardian of livestock, a beast of burden, a rescuer of lost people, a puller of carts and sleds, a friend, a hunter, a companion, an exercise mate, a guide for the blind and deaf, a contact with nature for urbanites, a way for city dwellers to meet people (the "dog-people," for example, in New York City), a source of friendship and company and solace for the old and lonely, a vehicle for penetrating the frightful shell surrounding the disturbed child, a source for the comfort of touch, and an inexhaustible wellspring of love.

Yet it is we who systematically violate this contract in the most essential ways, callously infringing upon the dog's rights to life and nature. The violation of the right to life is obvious. Each year we kill about 10 million healthy dogs in pounds and veterinarians' offices. We kill by barbiturates, decompression, carbon monoxide, shooting, electrocution. Millions more die of disease, starvation, and automobile accidents after they have been turned loose by owners. And the overwhelming majority of animals killed are not feral animals who have never had a home—this population would be reduced to insignificance after a few years of efficient animal control—but animals who have at one point been owned by a person.

Over the past four years I have worked closely with the people who run the humane society in my home city, as well as managers of humane societies and pounds across North America. Highly conscientious people, they have attempted to catalog the reasons people bring animals in to be euthanized. (Bringing an animal into a humane society or pound is tantamount to bringing them in to be killed. Very few will in fact be adopted.) Their results are echoed by veterinarians, who are also asked to put animals to sleep for extramedical reasons. People bring animals in to be killed because they are moving and do not want the trouble of traveling with a pet. People kill animals because they are moving to a place where it will be difficult to keep an animal. People kill animals because they are going on vacation and do not want to pay for boarding, and, anyway, one can always get another pet. People kill animals because their son or daughter is going away to college and cannot take care of it. People kill animals rather than attempting to place them in other homes, because "the animal could not bear to live without me." People kill animals because they cannot housebreak them, or train them not to jump on the furniture, or not to scratch or chew it. People kill animals because they have moved or redecorated and the animals no longer match the color scheme. People kill animals because the animals are not mean enough, or because they are too mean. People kill animals because they bark at strangers, or because they don't bark at strangers. People kill animals because the animal is getting old and can no longer jog with them. People kill animals because they feel themselves getting old and are afraid of dying before the animal. People kill animals because the semester is over and Mom and Dad would not appreciate a new dog. People kill animals because they only wanted their children to witness the "miracle of birth," and have no use for the puppies or kittens. People kill animals because they have heard that when Great Danes get old, they get mean. People kill animals because they are tired of them or because they want a new one. People kill animals because they are no longer puppies and kittens and are no longer cute. Clearly the legitimate reasons for violating animals' rights to life do not fall into these categories.

Equally intolerable from a moral point of view are our flagrant violations of the pet animals' right to live their lives in accordance with their natures — natures we have shaped. Sometimes these violations are the result of deliberate cruelty, as in the case of the sadistic individual who keeps a dog chained day and night. But most often, these violations grow out of ignorance and stupidity. The average person who acquires a dog or cat is worse than ignorant, worse because s/he is invariably infused with outrageously false information.

Consider some of the "common knowledge" about the natures of dogs and cats. Doberman pinscher's brains grow too large for their skulls and they go crazy. Cats suffocate babies. Dogs of the same sex will always fight if put together. A cat will always survive a fall. Big dogs should not be kept in city apartments. Purebred dogs are "better" than mongrels. The way to make a dog mean is to feed it gunpowder. Cats can't swim. Dogs and cats can't get along. The way to housebreak a dog is to hit it when it defecates in the house or to rub its nose in the excrement. If a dog is wagging its tail, it is friendly and won't bite. Slapping a dog on the nose is a good method of correction. Slapping a rolled up newspaper and startling the dog is a good method of correction. Cats cannot be trained. Castration or spaying of an animal removes aggression. And, of course, that time honored piece of folk wisdom, "You can't teach an old dog new tricks." These popular beliefs are, of course, false. To put it bluntly, the average person is either ignorant or misinformed about dog and cat behavior, training, biology, nutrition—in short, about the animal's nature. In some contexts this ignorance or misinformation is laughable, as when one man informed me that his dog is part bear, or a veterinary student informed me that Dobermans were mean because we had cropped their ears for generations, and that this resulted in hereditary ill temper. ("After all, how would you feel if someone cropped your ears? Pretty mean.") But most often the net result of this ignorance is a life for the animal where its basic nature is abused, thwarted, or ignored. Walk into a parking lot on a hot summer day and attend to the number of dogs left in closed cars without water or ventilation. ("He's just a small dog; there's plenty of air.") In point of fact, if the temperature inside the car reaches 105°—not at all unlikely given the greenhouse effect—the dog will suffer permanent brain damage within 15 minutes.

Or consider the claim mentioned above that one ought not keep a large dog in a city apartment, one of the few things that "everyone knows" when they go out to get a dog. Cognizant of that "fact," a family may decide to purchase a small poodle, with unfortunate consequences. The poodle, typically a frenetic, high-strung creature, will be miserable without constant exercise. They would very likely have been better off with a Great Dane, a phlegmatic dog which, despite its size, or perhaps because of it, tends to spend most of its time in a semicataleptic state. (In the case of our Dane my wife and I would call her periodically just to make sure she was still breathing. Generally we were lucky to exact one tail-thump in response.)

Veterinarians are excellent sources of information about the animal suffering engendered by human ignorance. All too often a veterinarian is asked to kill a dog, sometimes a puppy but more often an older dog, who is tearing up the house, or urinating on the bed. The owners have tried beating, yelling, caging; nothing has worked. They are shocked to learn that the dog, since it is a social animal, is lonely. Often the older dog has been played with every day for years by children who have now gone off to college. Often the dog has been accustomed to extraordinary attention from its mistress, who may suddenly have acquired a new boyfriend and has forgotten the dog's needs. Often the dog has been a child substitute for a young couple who now have a new baby and the dog is being ignored and is jealous.

Veterinarians are called upon almost daily to modify an animal's nature to suit an owner. Consider the case of the house-proud woman who has bought a cute kitten on a whim, oblivious to the fact that kittens climb, scratch things, exercise, or "sharpen" their claws on furniture. The "solution": declaw the animal and throw it outside in good weather. Unfortunately, the declawed animal is now devoid of natural defenses, and is likely to come home maimed, if at all. Or consider the case of the suburban couple who buy a dog, leave it outside at night, and then field complaints from neighbors that the dog barks. The "solution": surgically remove the voice box—a mutilation called debarking. This generally does not work, serving only to leave the animal with a grotesque honking noise. The American Kennel Club and similar organizations of dog and cat breed fanciers, are major culprits in perpetuating mutilations and distortions of animals' *telos,* through the "breed standards" they promulgate and perpetuate in dog and cat shows. If one wishes to win in these shows one must have a Doberman pinscher with cropped ears and docked tail; a Great Dane, Boxer, Boston bull terrier with cropped ears; a cocker spaniel, Old English sheepdog, poodle with docked tails.

In a related area mindless concern with standards that are purely esthetic or morphological results in perpetuation of genetic defects that cause much suffering in the dog. Concern with a certain shaped face and eye in the collie and Shetland sheepdog has led to a disease called "collie eye" or "sheltie eye," which can result in blindness. The breathing difficulties and heart problems of bulldogs are genetically and physiologically linked to the selection for foreshortened faces. There is some evidence that German shepherd aggressiveness, much prized by trainers and the military, is genetically linked to hip dysplasia. The Irish setter has been bred with an exclusive concern for esthetics to the point of imbecility. (It is sometimes said of these dogs that "they cannot find themselves at the end of a leash.") Manx cats, bred for taillessness, suffer from severe spinal defects. Dachshunds suffer from genetically based spinal diseases that result in paralysis; and they tend to have diabetes and Cushing's disease. Dalmatians get bladder stones, apparently as a result of genetic linkage with coat color. In dalmatians and Australian shepherds, coat color is linked with hereditary deafness. Siamese cats are bred for cross-eyes. Silver-colored collies suffer from Grey Collie syndrome, a situation where their white blood cell count cyclically falls, and they become susceptible to infection. They also become susceptible to digestive, reproductive, skeletal, and ocular problems. Boxers have by far the greatest incidence of every sort of cancers of all dog breeds. (In fact, more than one hundred diseases of dogs are of genetic origin; that is, perpetuated by irresponsible breeding.) In short, not only do we *ignore* relevant aspects of our animals' natures, we also systematically *destroy* these natures through breeding for traits that appeal to us, without regard for the effect of these traits on the animals' lives.

Other examples of violations of animal nature are manifest. Through our own failure to understand and respect dogs, train them properly, and understand their psychology, we tranquilize our pets, cage them in tiny cages for hours, chain them, muzzle them, beat them, use choke collars. Instead of using the dog's natural protectiveness of home and master, we create instant attack dogs through brutal training methods, dogs who bite anything that moves, including the owner. Many of these dogs are hairtrigger weapons, primed by stimulus and response and sold to people who know nothing about dogs and who think that by plunking down $2,000 they have bought respect and loyalty. Many of these dogs, especially those male dogs trained by men and sold to women, are subsequently destroyed for being "uncontrollable." Our failure to know little if anything about the dog's biology or behavior results in people buying any dog as long as it is "cute," which in turn results in unscrupulous puppy mills that turn out inferior animals under appalling conditions for profit. Pet stores often neglect and abuse their animals. Our lack of understanding of animals' nutritional and biological needs results in myriad medical problems that arise from poor diet, overfeeding, and lack of exercise. Our use of animals as extensions of ourselves rather than ends in themselves results in the encouragement of behavior that is unnatural or neurotic — begging, limping for sympathy, whining for attention. Our inability to understand the animal results in an inability to train it, which in turn leads to dogs who chase cars and are killed or maimed in traffic accidents (or engender accidents that harm humans); dogs who chase joggers and are maced; dogs who are euthanized because they nip children. Our failure to confine our animals results in their being shot by farmers, being run over, becoming pregnant indiscriminately or at an age that stunts their development, being unwanted because of overproduction, and doing damage to lawns and gardens. We have increased the danger of disease through wholesale deposit of excrement in the cities. Worst of all, our neglect has led to pack formation of wild dogs in the rural areas of our country.

We are far indeed from respecting the fundamental rights of pet animals. Our laws mirror our individual irresponsibility. The laws see pet animals as private property; anyone can acquire an animal, and usually as many as they wish. Only the anticruelty laws "protect" the animals; these are rarely enforced and in some states require proof of malicious intent, required not so much to protect the animals as to weed out sadistic individuals who might harm humans.

Thus we can conclude that we are dealing with a morally intolerable situation, all the more so because our legal system and our educational system do nothing to break the cycle. We need to provide laws to protect these creatures, laws that make it harder to own — and destroy — an animal. We must furthermore — and here veterinarians are obliged to lead the way — educate people as to animal needs and rights.

Let us be aware that grief for pet animals is more than just an overflow for draining emotion. It is also a springboard for awakening our moral concern for the millions of creatures who have intrinsic value, whose lives are wasted and twisted at our hands, and yet for whom no tears are shed.

REFERENCE

Rollin, B. E. 1981. *Animal rights and human morality.* Buffalo, N.Y.: Prometheus.

2

Pet Animals
and Human Well-being

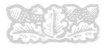

M . W . F O X

SEVERAL OF THE VARIOUS KINDS of human/animal relationships that Kellert (1980) describes have been detailed in another review of people's relationships with their pets (Fox 1980). From these studies, it may be concluded that similar percepts, concepts, needs, and values underlie people's attitudes toward wild animals and that these also influence their relationship with one or more companion animals. However, it must be remembered that these attitudes are not always consistent: Thus, while a family may enjoy eating roast duck, it would be unthinkable to consider killing and eating the pet duck that once was the children's Easter duckling.

Similarly, for emotional reasons, Europeans do not consider the dog as a source of food. For the British, eating dog is akin perhaps to cannibalism, while for the Chinese it is a delicacy. I have met farmers who have been unable to slaughter, or to eat after slaughtering, animals the family became attached to. It is not surprising therefore that people experience a sense of loss when such animals die. When the same animals are objects of sheer utility, however, few if any constraints are applied in treating them as mere objects. This phenomenon is a source of widespread institutionalized exploitation and covert animal cruelty (Fox 1980).

A person's emotional reaction to the loss of a pet will therefore be determined primarily by that person's degree of involvement with that animal (particularly in terms of dependence and attendant values and perceptions) as well as by cultural influences. The reaction will be a composite of many and sometimes conflicting feelings and concepts, including *guilt or remorse* ("I should have saved her"); hurt redirected as *anger* ("the veterinarian was dumb" or "it was a stupid truck driver"); and *denial* of responsibility ("the owner should not have let the animal roam free and get run over").

In more extreme cases, the owner may believe that the animal will return (*wishful thinking*) when it has been lost and missing for weeks; or that it is not really dead, even after having seen it die (*magical thinking* or *psychotic delusion*). Many pet owners will say they have no intention of ever getting another pet, a reaction to emotional loss that is *protective* in that they do not wish to go through the same hurt again. In contrast others may get an immediate replacement, sometimes of the same sex and breed in order to help overcome the sense of loss. I have met owners who believe that their deceased pet might be reincarnated in their new one (*mystical-magical thinking*).

Parents may encounter difficulties explaining the death of the pet to their children, more so if the parents have difficulty coping with their own grief and sense of loss. Such remarks as "it was only an animal after all, so why get upset" or "never mind, we'll get another pet soon" are meant to lighten the child's hurt, but they only make things worse and make the parents seem insensitive. The frustration and anger the child feels over the loss of the pet may then be redirected toward the parents.

While pet cemeteries have been ridiculed, they can provide an important function, especially for families who have no backyard to bury their pet in. Ritual burial is part of the individuation and self-healing from the loss of a loved one, as well as a symbol of respect and appreciation.

How much a person reacts to the death of the pet in terms of losing a companion, a responsive and affectionate being that is valued in and for itself, may be variously proportional to the degree of personal investment, attachment, and dependence upon the animal. Do people who primarily relate to and value their pets in and for themselves, suffer more, or less, or differently, from those who have far more emotional involvement, dependence, and anthropomorphic projection and identification with their pets? Conversely how do pets of these two extreme forms of owner relationship (need dependency and transpersonal) (Fox 1980) react to owner loss through death or separation? The close bond that can be established between man and animal is a remarkable illustration of interspecies communication (Boone 1956; Fox 1980b). While the therapeutic value of companion animals is becoming more widely recognized, the educational benefits should not be overlooked as a major contributing factor to overall human well-being (Fox 1980). The absence of animals during early formative years could well impoverish the development of human consciousness (Shepard 1978). Worse, perhaps, in the absence of early socialization, affectional ties, and other experiences with animals, a child may well mature to be indifferent toward animals. Such indifference is a major contributing factor to the widespread institutionalized exploitation of animals by contemporary society. It may also cut humanity off from its biological roots, which would surely jeopardize both the quality of human experience and the quality of the environment.

There are people today who mourn the passing of the condor, the sperm whale, and the wolf in ways not unlike others who might grieve over the loss of their pet. However, species extinction is a very different order of magnitude, and while empathy plays an important part in animal welfare and in the prevention of cruelty, there may be less empathy and more identification intrinsically with regard to the plight of endangered species. This identification and concern may stem from a subconscious or intuitive feeling that we are all part of the same creation, of One Earth One Mind (Fox 1980c).

To some extent I agree with Shepard (1978) that a manufactured toy pet, such as a toy poodle, may not be the optimal creature to give a child a sense of the "otherness" of animals and a respect for their intrinsic nature and value in and for themselves. However, the toy poodle need not be perceived and treated as a cuddly windup toy or "doglet": much depends upon the attitudes and values expressed by the child's parents. A wild animal might be considered a better learning experience for the child, but to raise one as a pet or keep it captive would be a gross misperception and probably more damaging to the child's developing sense of values than keeping a toy poodle as a pet "toy."

There are many anecdotes of how cats, dogs, and other animals react to human or animal companion loss (Burton 1978; Fox 1978), notably "depression," which includes reduced physical activity, disinterest in surroundings and people; withdrawal and cessation of usual daily routines; and, occasionally, anorexia. Other signs of loss may include mournful howling, pacing, searching, and waiting with unusual anticipation for the owner's return at the usual time. Anecdotes are also told of cats and dogs that have reacted suddenly and without any obvious foreknowledge to the death of a companion animal. For example, a Siamese cat in Philadelphia began to call loudly and incessantly at 10 A.M. the morning after the evening before when its companion, an aged German shepherd, was rushed to the veterinary hospital. The veterinarian called at 11 A.M. that morning to tell the owner that the dog had died on the operating table at 10 A.M. The owner had already been prepared for this loss by her cat's acting so strangely, but how did the cat know?

Various metaphysical, or what I prefer to call *metabiological* theories, can be elaborated to explain such phenomena, but without very carefully designed and controlled laboratory or field studies, we may well remain forever on the threshold of understanding. How a dog or cat can "psi-trail" and locate its family hundreds of miles away in a place it has never before been (Fox 1972) is another question for future research. It is a well-documented phenomenon, and is related to how an animal behaves when separated from loved ones. Can an animal sense a difference between owner loss from separation (geographically) and from death? Studies on separation depression in infant primates (Sackett 1968) show similar reaction sequences to those described in parentally deprived human infants. In pets, too, somewhat similar symptoms are seen when the animal is left at a boarding kennel or is hospitalized, or when its owner or a companion animal in the house dies or leaves for an extended period. Captive animals of various species also manifest a variety of emotional reactions, ranging from self-mutilation to anorexia and depression following loss of or separation from a cage mate (Meyer-Holtzapfel 1968).

There may well be a common thread linking "psi-trailing" with suprasensory awareness of the death of a companion, an animal's reaction to the death of its owner, and vice versa. Within the complex psychophysical, metabiological phenomenon of intra- and interspecies affectional bonding, there may be a subjective element of experience or affect that is beyond the realm of objective scientific elucidation. Yet its analysis may be what contemporary, reductionistic, and mechanistic science needs to restore its validity and scholarship.

The science of animal welfare (Dawkins 1980) and of a cognitive ethology (Griffin 1977) is slowly dawning, and is characterized by an interdisciplinary, holistic (nonlinear) approach to the questions of animal well-being and their affective, subjective states. This is more a "break into" than a "break through," and its purpose is to understand animal behavior for its own sake rather than for sheer intellectual curiosity or utility. It represents, I believe, a radical departure from the usual motivational and cognitive approach of scientific inquiry, which has traditionally been based upon Baconian utopianism, Cartesianism, dominionism, and hubris (Fox 1980; Morris and Fox 1978). The approach now is less humanocentric and more animal centered or zoocentric and ecocentric, and certainly less mechanistically reductionistic. It is this kind of approach that characterizes the present discussion of the dynamics of the pet-owner bond and of the short- and long-term consequences of the bond being broken. What is the nature of this bond? What behavioral, physiological, psychological, and cultural parameters influence its strength or intensity? How is it expressed, experienced, and shared by reciprocal parties and how are interspecies barriers in communication and needs dealt with? An understanding of these questions could mean a greater understanding of what is meant by health, wholeness, love, healing, bereavement, and affect-dependence, with obvious enhancement in the practice of animal and human medicine. Bakan (1968) reviews many studies that show how stress associated with the sudden loss of a companion or loved one correlates with an increased incidence of various diseases, including certain forms of cancer in humans. A greater understanding of "ease," of the general sense of well-being and associated health that correlate with strong supportive affectional ties with others, and the "dis-ease" and sickness that correlate with either the breaking of a strong affectional tie or the complete absence of it in a person's life will be promising and challenging avenues for future research.

REFERENCES

Bakan, D. 1968. *Disease, pain and sacrifice: Toward a psychology of suffering.* Boston: Beacon.

Burton, M. 1978. *Just like an animal.* New York: Scribner.

Boone, J. A. 1956. *Kinship with all life.* New York: Harper and Row.

Dawkins, M. 1980. *Animal suffering: The science of animal welfare.* London: Chapman and Hall.

Fogle, B., ed. 1981. *Interrelations between people and pets.* Springfield, Ill.: Charles C Thomas.

Fox, M. W. 1972. *Understanding your dog.* New York: Coward, McCann and Geoghegan.

──────. 1978. *Understanding your pet.* New York: Coward, McCann and Geoghegan.

──────. 1980. *Returning to Eden: Animal rights and human responsibility.* New York: Viking.

──────. 1980b. *The soul of the wolf.* Boston: Little, Brown.

──────. 1980c. *One earth one mind.* New York: Coward, McCann and Geoghegan.

Griffin, D. 1977. *The question of animal awareness.* New York: Rockefeller University Press.

Kellert, S. R. 1980. American attitudes toward and knowledge of animals: An update. *International Journal for the Study of Animal Problems* 1:87–119.

Meyer-Holtzapfel, M. 1968. Abnormal behavior in animals. In *Abnormal behavior in animals,* ed. M. W. Fox. Philadelphia: W. B. Saunders.

Morris, R. K., and M. W. Fox, eds. 1978. *On the fifth day: Animal rights and human ethics.* Washington, D.C.: Acropolis.

Sackett, G. P. 1968. Abnormal behavior in laboratory-reared Rhesus monkeys. In *Abnormal behavior in animals,* ed. M. W. Fox. Philadelphia: W. B. Saunders.

Shepard, P. 1978. *Thinking animals.* New York: Viking.

3

Health Consequences
of Pet Ownership

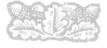

ERIKA FRIEDMANN, AARON A. KATCHER,
SUE A. THOMAS, JAMES J. LYNCH

THE LOSS OF A PET may affect the owner's health through two mechanisms: the grief response, and the loss of the health benefits provided by the pet. The loss of these benefits certainly can result in a loss of well-being and a diminution of every aspect of the owner's health.

Our research into the health benefits of pet ownership began with a study of the social, psychological, and physiological factors that affected the one-year survival of coronary heart disease patients. In our study of 92 white patients who had been admitted to a large university hospital for coronary heart disease, only 3 of the 53 pet owners died within the first year after admission, while 11 of the 39 people who did not own pets died in this same period. Since we recognized that keeping dogs may require more work than keeping other pets, we felt that by including dog owners in our analysis, we might actually be including people who were in better health. Thus we eliminated dog owners from our comparison. Yet a still significant difference in survival appeared, independent of the physiological severity of the illness, between those who owned pets but did not own dogs (0 out of 10 died), and the non–pet owners.

Most importantly, the effect of pet ownership was not present only in people who were socially isolated. It was independent of marital status and access to social support from other people (Friedmann et al. 1978; 1980a). These research findings suggest that pets may have important effects on the lives of adults—independent of and supplementary to the companionship of other people.

Thus we have asked, How can pets benefit people's health? We have identified seven functions of companion animals that could increase longevity and decrease morbidity of healthy adults. The functions that would be expected to have a positive influence on health are: (1) companionship, (2) something to care for, (3) something to keep one busy, (4) something to touch and fondle, (5) a relaxing focus of attention, (6) safety, and (7) exercise. The first three—companionship, something to care for, and something to keep one busy—act to decrease depression and loneliness. Anxiety and sympathetic nervous system arousal are decreased through the second three functions: something to touch and fondle, a relaxing focus of attention, and safety. The final function, providing an impetus for exercise, helps maintain physical fitness (Friedmann et al. 1980b; Katcher 1981; Katcher and Friedmann 1980). We will consider these functions and the experimental evidence for their potential health value.

Abundant evidence suggests that the companionship provided by a pet can both reduce the frequency of serious disease and prolong life. A large and consistent body of evidence indicates that single, divorced, and widowed individuals have higher disease rates and die earlier than married persons (Clayton et al. 1971; Kraus and Lilienfeld 1959; Lynch 1977; Parkes 1964). If a pet can provide companionship, it should be able to decrease the pathological effects of social isolation and loneliness. In a small study of the health benefits of pet ownership, Mugford and M'Comiskey (1975) placed budgerigars with 12 pensioners and begonias with 12 others. They reported improved health in those receiving birds 5 months after their introduction. Health was assessed using symptom and mood questionnaires.

Unfortunately, there are no large-scale studies of differences in mortality and morbidity rates of people who do and do not keep pets. The closest approximation of such a study was our investigation of coronary heart disease patient survival (Friedmann et al. 1978; Friedmann et al. 1980a).

Although it is important to demonstrate the strength of the companionship provided by a pet through epidemiological studies of health, it is also valuable to study the transactions that structure the bonds between people and their pets. Katcher has presented evidence for the important role of the pet in the family and described some of the transactions beween people and their pets (1981). Although almost everyone believes that pets provide companionship, demographic data on pet ownership indicate that the rate of pet ownership is highest among families with children and lowest among the most socially isolated segment of our population, the elderly (Christensen 1978; Schneider and Vaida 1975). This is paradoxically true despite the fact that many elderly individuals use animals for social companionship and form close interdependent relationships with their pets. In some instances they depend on their pets as their sole source of companionship.

As well as directly providing companionship, pets can also act as a bridge to facilitate meeting other adults, especially in impersonal areas, such as city streets, apartment house hallways, and elevators. Dr. S. A. Corson has used pets to facilitate interactions among residents of homes for the aged (Corson et al. 1977).

As a consequence of old age in American society, one loses both the opportunity and means to care for others. Often depression and loss of self-esteem, consequent to feeling useless, occur much earlier in life. When people feel useless, or when they feel a loss of reciprocity in their relationships with others, they retreat from social contacts and aggravate their isolation. The evidence already cited as to the longevity of married persons suggest that the positive effect of marriage on health is partially due to caring for one another. Social isolation results in both a lack of companionship and a lack of people to care for. It may be that caring for another person facilitates a pattern of psychoendocrine organization that results in a greater resistance to disease. For example, depression, which is associated with an unwillingness to care for others and to form close social relationships, results in psychoendocrine responses that increase the probability of disease and death (de la Fuente 1979; Tiger 1979).

Pets can stimulate the same kind of caring response evoked by children and adults. In a study of the way people pet animals in public places, many of the gestures used resemble those used to fondle and care for young children (Katcher et al. 1979; Katcher et al. 1983a).

A pet can also act as a transitional object (Winnicot 1953), even late in life, by helping a person transfer affection to others. Older people who have been depressed because of the loss of a relative or friend can learn to love others again through first learning to love and care for a pet.

The importance of contact comfort in the development of infants and young children has been documented extensively. Infants who are deprived of touch do not develop normally, and in severe instances may fail to thrive, and die (Klaus and Kennel 1976; Spitz 1945). Older infants and young children are very aggressive in seeking touch from their parents. There is a growing awareness that touch is an important means of displaying affection in young adult life. Little is known about the role of touch in older adults. It is known that human touch has powerful effects on the cardiovascular system. Even patients who were paralyzed with curare while being treated in a shock trauma unit showed dramatic responses to human touch (Lynch et al. 1974; Lynch et al. 1977).

It is not unreasonable to infer that touch acts in part by decreasing sympathetic arousal. Touch then can act as an antianxiety agent and can decrease the probability of progression in conditions that are worsened by constant emotional arousal (hypertension, stroke, diabetes mellitus). Our study of people greeting and petting their pets suggests that interacting with a pet may decrease the anxiety and sympathetic nervous system responses associated with moderately stressful situations (Friedmann et al. 1979; Katcher et al. 1983b).

While pets are an important source of contact comfort for adults and children, there have been few serious investigations of the way people pet their pets. Three important findings resulted from our study of how people pet their pets in a public place. First, there was no difference between men and women in the frequency, amount, and kind of touching. This is surprising because men are stereotyped as being less able than women to express affection with touch in public (Goffman 1976). Apparently dogs are an approved means for men to express and receive affection in public. Second, there was no quantitative difference in people's tactile interactions with small, medium, and large dogs. This finding suggests that all breeds of dogs provide an outlet for touch (Friedmann et al. 1980b; Katcher 1981; Katcher et al. 1983a; Lynch 1977). Our third finding was the observation that tactile interactions with pets take two forms: engaged and idle. In engaged petting the person's attention is focused on the animal; while during idle petting the person's attention is focused elsewhere. Idle petting resembles the absent-minded fondling of a child while attention is focused elsewhere. (Friedmann et al. 1980b; Katcher 1981; Katcher et al. 1979; Katcher et al. 1983a). Idly fondling a pet can provide reverie and relaxation in a public place.

More information is needed about the ways older people express affection through handling their pets and the importance of affection in their lives. Certainly for many isolated people, young and old, a pet may be the only source of contact comfort.

Americans believe it is important to keep busy. This attitude is one of the reasons retirement is such a mixed blessing. After retirement people who have always had something to do suddenly find themselves with nothing to do. This lack of meaningful activity can engender a feeling of uselessness and depression.

The presence of an animal, especially one that demands attention from the owner, provides a stimulus for a daily routine. This can prevent the disorganization in time that may occur after retirement when the time orientation of workaday life is removed.

There is also direct evidence that keeping busy may have important positive effects on the longevity of older people. In a National Institutes of Health study of healthy older men, a large number of physiological, social, and psychological variables were correlated with 10-year survival. Only two variables were strong predictors of survival: not smoking and a complex routine of varied daily activities (Goffman 1976; Libow 1963). This study did not consider pet ownership. However, it can be deduced that the presence of a pet can add to the interest, complexity, and variability of a daily routine.

Animals can provide a relaxing focus of attention. Personal experience and psychological research have shown that a gentle focus of attention can be comforting and can draw attention away from private and perhaps painful thoughts toward the neutral world outside. This type of direction of attention toward the environment has been observed to be an important means of reducing excitement and sympathetic arousal. When anxious subjects are asked to attend to instructions, watch a display of lights, or listen to music, heart rate falls and palmar sweating decreases (Lacey et al. 1963).

Remaining silent and listening to the unvoiced repetition of a word or syllable may be the basis for the relaxation effects of transcendental meditation. Such meditative exercise may be a complex way of attaining a state of relaxation by focusing attention away from possibly disturbing private thoughts toward gentle relaxing thoughts like those provided by watching the motions of a tank of tropical fish, a few hamsters in a cage, a cat, or a bird.

For the urban elderly crime in the streets is a personal experience rather than a political slogan. The fear of being injured is often a significant factor in decreasing their ability to use facilities of the city and increasing their isolation from friends and relatives. Older people may also be forced from their independent residences by fear of being attacked while alone. Fear also increases depression in the aged by making them feel trapped and helpless. Anything that decreases fear and depression is likely to have direct beneficial effects on psychological, social, and physiological health. Sebkova (1977) showed that the presence of a pet may alter perception of anxiety in a complex environment. She found that persons present in a psychological laboratory were less anxious when her dog was present in the lab and in their homes, and that the subjects paid more attention to the dog in a laboratory situation than in their homes. Thus the presence of a pet may make a situation seem less threatening. Future research will be directed toward discovering if there is also a lowering of sympathetic arousal when a pet is present. A dog can decrease fear and make a neighborhood feel safer, thereby increasing an individual's willingness to move about freely. It is known that people feel safer with a dog. It is not known how much safer people are in the presence of a dog. Improved police statistics are needed on the frequency of muggings and break-ins experienced by people with and without dogs. In particular, it is important to know the extent to which the size of the dog is a factor in its safety value. Whether it is the potential bite or the bark that is the deterrent must be determined. If small dogs are as effective protection as large ones, people can be encouraged to own smaller dogs, which they can manage and afford more easily.

While jogging seems to be the current fashion, there is no definite evidence that it is more beneficial to health than walking. Dogs provide a stimulus for walking and, in some instances, a reminder to keep going out when motivation falters. The animal provides a stimulus for regular repetition of exercises and an interesting source of stimulation during exercise. The dog walker finds it easier to meet and talk to others and is rewarded by the animal's pleasure in being taken out.

Until recently, a large body of anecdotal information and a strong folk belief suggested that pets were good for you, especially if "you" were a child. However, there was no research to support the hypothesis that pets have important effects on the lives of healthy adults. The evidence presented suggests that pets can function to improve their owner's well-being. Thus the loss of a pet could have a significant impact on the owner's health. The effects of the loss may be especially acute for elderly isolated individuals who have minimal support from other sources.

REFERENCES

Christensen, A. M. 1978. *City of Toronto pet survey.* Toronto: Toronto Humane Society.

Clayton, P. J., J. A. Halikas, and W. Maurice. 1971. The bereavement of widowhood. *Diseases of the Nervous System* 32:597–604.

Corson, S. A., E. O. Corson, and R. Gunsett. 1977. The socializing role of pet animals in nursing homes: An experiment in nonverbal communication therapy. In *Society stress and disease: Aging and old age.* Oxford: Oxford University Press.

de la Fuente, J. R. 1979. Endocrine changes in depressive illness. *Psychiatric Annals* 9:37–50.

Friedmann, E., S. A. Thomas, A. H. Katcher, and M. Noctor. 1978. Pet ownership and coronary heart disease patient survival. *Circulation* 58:II-168 (abstract).

Friedmann, E., A. H. Katcher, D. Meislich, and M. Goodman. 1979. Physiological response of people to petting their pets. *American Zoologist* 19:327 (abstract).

Friedmann, E., A. H. Katcher, J. J. Lynch, and S. A. Thomas. 1980a. Animal companions and one year survival of patients after discharge from a coronary care unit. *Public Health Reports* 95:307–12.

––––––. 1980b. Potential health benefits of companion animals. Paper presented at the annual Scientific Sessions of the American Public Health Association, Detroit (October).

Goffman, E. 1976. Gender advertisements. *Studies in the Anthropology of Visual Communication* 3:65–154.

Katcher, A. H. 1981. Form and function in the human-companion animal bond. In *Interrelations between people and pets*, ed. B. Fogel. Springfield, Ill.: Charles C Thomas.

Katcher, A. H., and E. Friedmann. 1980. Potential health value of pet ownership. *Compendium on Continuing Education for the Practicing Veterinarian.* 2:117–21.

Katcher, A. H. et al. 1983a. Men, women, and dogs. In press.

Katcher, A. H. et al. 1983b. Social interaction and blood pressure: Influence of animal companions. In press.

Katcher, A. H., L. Goodman, and E. Friedmann. 1979. Human-pet interactions. *American Zoologist.* 19:326 (abstract).

Klaus, M. K., and J. H. Kennell. 1976. *Maternal-infant bonding: The impact of early separation or loss on family development.* St. Louis: C. V. Mosby.

Kraus, A. S., and A. Lilienfeld. 1959. Some epidemiologic aspects of the high mortality rate in the young widowed group. *Journal of Chronic Diseases* 10:207–17.

Lacey, J. I. et al. 1963. Situational determinants and behavioral correlates of autonomic response patterns. In *Expression of the emotions in man,* ed. P. J. Knapp. New York: International Universities Press.

Libow, L. S. 1963. Medical investigation of the process of aging. In *Human aging: A biological and behavioral study,* (PHS) 98-6, ed. J. E. Biren et al. Washington, D.C.: GPO.

Lynch, J. J. 1977. *The broken heart: The medical consequences of loneliness.* New York: Basic Books.

Lynch, J. J. et al. 1974. The effects of human contact on cardiac arrhythmia in coronary care patients. *Journal of Nervous and Mental Disease* 158:88–98.

Lynch, J. J. et al. 1977. Human contact and cardiac arrhythmia in a coronary care unit. *Psychosomatic Medicine* 39:188.

Mugford, R. A., and I. G. M'Comiskey. 1975. Some recent work on the psychotherapeutic value of cage birds with old people. In *Pet animals and society,* ed. R. S. Anderson. London: Bailliere-Tindall.

Parkes, C. M. 1964. Effects of bereavement on physical and mental health: A study of the medical records of widows. *British Medical Journal* 2:274–79.

Schneider, R., and M. L. Vaida. 1975. Survey of canine and feline populations: Alameda and Contra Costa Counties, California, 1970. *Journal of the American Veterinary Medical Association* 166:481–86.

Sebkova, J. 1977. Anxiety levels as affected by the presence of a dog. Master's thesis, University of Lancaster, Lancaster, England.

Spitz, R. A. 1945. Hospitalism: An inquiry into the genesis of psychiatric conditions in early childhood. *Psychoanalytic Study of the Child* 1:53–74.

Tiger, L. 1979. *Optimism: The biology of hope.* New York: Simon and Schuster.

Winnicot, D. W. 1953. Transitional objects and transitional phenomena. *International Journal of Psychoanalysis* 24:88–97.

Youmans, E. G., and M. Yarrow. Aging and social adaptation: A longitudinal study of healthy old men. In *Human aging II: An eleven year follow-up biomedical and behavioral study,* (HSM) 70-9037, ed. S. Granick, and R. D. Patterson. Washington, D.C.: GPO.

4

Nonconventional
Human/Companion Animal Bonds

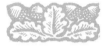

JAMES M. HARRIS

SURVEYS OF VETERINARY PRACTICES in the United States have
shown that 50 million animal contacts are made by companion
animal veterinary practitioners each year. With two humans accompanying each animal visit, 100 million human contacts are
made yearly. Surveys also have found that 4 percent of animal
patient visits involve the death or euthanasia of the patient. With
12,000 active companion animal practitioners, the average number
of natural or induced mortalities is 166 per practitioner per year
(3.2 cases per week). It is not uncommon for a busy or specialty
practice to have one or more fatalities each practice day. Each of
these has, with few exceptions, some degree of client grief and
emotional turmoil.

Clients who have nonconventional bonds with their companion
animals often exhibit more pronounced and intense emotional response at that time. Keddie (1977) observed:

Those who insist on a special relationship with their dog or cat put themselves at a risk from a mental health point of view. In cases where such
over-dependence on a pet does exist, there is likely to be a sharp reaction
on the part of the owner when the pet dies or has to be "put to sleep."

Clients who have special relationships with their companion
animals generally have a higher number of veterinary service con-

tacts per animal per year. They tend also to be more attentive to their pets' physical and emotional states and, needless to say, are more anxious than clients with conventional companion animal bonds when there is illness, trauma, a guarded-to-poor prognosis, terminal states, or death.

All veterinary practitioners have some clients with nonconventional bonds. The veterinarian who shows understanding, compassion, concern, and support for clients as well as for patients, and who has a well-developed "bedside manner," has a disproportionately high number of these clients. Word of mouth recommendations by these clients, and colleague referrals further increase the number of this type of client seen by these practitioners.

The successful practitioner-client relationship is usually a most complicated interchange. This certainly is the case with many clients who have nonconventional bonds with their companion animals. Client trust and confidence are essential for success. If the relationship is successful, the companion animal receives quality lifetime care and medical supervision, the client is comfortable in the professional setting, and this good relationship continues with existing pets or future pets acquired after the death of a particular companion animal.

But this is not always the case. Mrs. P, a woman in her sixties, married, all children grown and successful, has some fifteen cats in her home. Over a period of two to three years she had presented many of these cats for treatment. Since she had both feline infectious peritonitis virus and feline leukovirus in her cat population, the frequency of illness and visits was high, and typically one or more cats was seriously or terminally ill. Because of the frequency of her visits she was sometimes seen by an associate in the practice. Rapport with Mrs. P was excellent until one day she presented a moribund, anemic, FeLV+ cat for euthanasia. The associate practitioner provided this service for her with great skill in her presence as she wished. Until this time, other cats had been euthanized without incident and she expressed thanks for our kindness and understanding. On this particular occasion, the patient took two postinjection reflex gasps after cardiac arrest. The client paid her bill and left without comment. A few days later, I phoned her to express my condolences and give reassurance that the correct decision had been made. She thanked me and then announced she would not be coming back to us for service. No, she was not displeased with us. She had been advised in the past about agonal reflexes, since she always requested to be present during euthanasia and we wanted to prepare her in the event that it occurred. Now she felt that she could never come to the hospital again without remembering "those two gasps."

I hope she has found another understanding practitioner. It has been my experience that many clients switch veterinarians after the death of a companion animal if they acquire a new pet, and continue to do this so long as they have pets and do not run out of veterinarians.

Other health professionals do not always appreciate the deep loss felt by humans at the death of a companion animal. A psychiatrist acquaintance once had a patient arrive for her hour in a most agitated state. When asked why she was so upset and crying, she stated that her cat, Fluffy, had died that morning. "Oh," said the therapist, "I am sorry to hear that." "But you do not realize how close Fluffy was to me," said the patient. "She was just like my own fur and bones."

The veterinarian can and should reach out to clients at times of grief. Words of comfort, a phone call, a letter, a card, or "holding a hand," are all appropriate actions and need to be selected for the particular case.

Mr. S, a construction worker, married, with children in their teens, had a yellow Labrador retriever/golden retriever crossbred dog who accompanied him wherever he went. The dog even climbed ladders and spent days at work with his master on construction scaffolding. The dog was presented for examination in June in apparent good health. In July, the dog became profoundly ill and in August a diagnosis of thoracic malignancy was made. While viewing the radiographs, discussing the prognosis, and finally requesting euthanasia, Mr. S started to cry. "Just a simple dog for simple folk," he said through his tears. I put my arm around this 6-foot, 3-inch, 200-plus pound man, and, a little wet-eyed myself, said, "No, a special dog for very special people." He now has a new puppy who, he hopes, will be climbing ladders soon.

Miss G, a spinster, retired, in her seventies, acquired a 4-year-old beagle when a friend died. Miss G had promised to care for the animal in the event his mistress died. She wanted to go home to Scotland to spend her last years, but kept putting it off because she was apprehensive about the dog's ability to make the trip. When she went and took the dog, he was more than 11 years old. The dog died in quarantine one week before the end of the 6-month period and one week past his twelfth birthday. Heartbroken, Miss G wrote:

I have the saddest of news. Dear wee Dukie passed away on September 9th. I can't believe it. I'm sure you must know how I feel. I wish I had never come away. Dear Duke, used to so much love and comfort! He was so upset when I left him at the kennel. I thought it better not to visit so I never saw him alive again. It's breaking my heart. Why, Dr. Harris, did it happen so near his time for freedom and eight days after his twelfth birthday? If he had only died in his own house with me beside him. But he must have wondered where I had gone and why I had left him. I'll never forgive myself. . . . I just know my pet has gone and left me very lonely and sad. . . .

A letter and a phone call from me when I was in Great Britain helped to reduce her feelings of guilt and sadness, although she still expresses grief over her loss.

Mrs. W, retired, a French immigrant in her seventies, had had a white dove for 5 years. The bird flew out of the house and was severely mauled by a cat. Most of the crop was destroyed with much trauma to the neck, making prognosis very guarded. The client asked us to attempt "to save my special friend." A number of surgeries were performed, and the client was most helpful with her at-home nursing and feeding. A month later, the bird was euthanized because of nonhealing of the crop and surrounding tissue and a profound decline in condition. Knowing that all possible had been done medically and surgically, and receiving a phone call from me the following day, greatly eased this client's grief.

The death of a companion animal to pediatric clients can be very upsetting. R, a 9-year-old patient at a special center for emotionally handicapped children, came to school one morning expressing great guilt over the death of his cat. He was sure he had killed the animal. When the social worker called me, I suggested that if she, the boy, and the cat's remains came for an appointment, I might be able to help. The child's parents were contacted, readily agreed, refrigerated the remains and scheduled an appointment time for the following day. I discussed the case with the child and discovered that he had found the cat already dead under a bush in his front yard. I proposed to do a necropsy to determine the cause of death and the boy agreed to this. Simple surface examination revealed that the cat had been struck by a car and had either been knocked from the road to the yard under the bush or had run that far after having been struck, only to die there from massive head injuries. When this was shown to the child, he was greatly relieved.

Occasionally, the client works things out in spite of the practitioner's efforts. Miss C, a single woman with an 8-year-old Tibetan terrier with terminal malignant disease, presented the dog in a terminal coma for evaluation. The dog was brought to the examination room wrapped in a pair of her pajamas and a robe. Euthanasia was performed, and she requested that we wrap the dog in her garments. The client wanted to arrange for cremation and requested that we keep the remains overnight. I told her that I would comply with her wishes and refrigerate the remains until she came for them. When Miss C returned the following morning, I was off duty. My staff reported that she showed great concern about her pajamas and robe, asking where they were. The technician and receptionist did not know and told her I would call her later in the day. When the box was brought to her, she touched it and finding it cold, moved a couple of feet away from it. Despite repeated efforts by staff to help her and talk to her, she sat there in silence for over an hour. Finally, she took the box and left. When I reached her by phone in the late afternoon, she said she wanted to launder her garments. I reminded her of her wish to have her beloved pet wrapped in them. She said, "Oh, yes, but I just thought you would wrap him up for a few hours." Then she advised me that the box with the remains had been cremated that afternoon. She sounded very sad, both for the loss of her dog and her pajamas and robe. I was just about to express my sympathies on the loss of her pet and reassure her that she had made a proper, humane decision when she said, "Isn't it significant that my dog died the day the Dalai Lama arrived in San Francisco!? He was a Tibetan dog, you know." I have since added the Dalai Lama to my list of practice aids.

Nonconventional bonds are many, varied, and occur in the variety of client populations seen by veterinary practitioners. Pediatric clients to geriatric clients, singles and couples, straights and gays, large and small family groups—all have such bonds with animals. Since most companion animals have life expectancies much shorter than their human stewards, we must be prepared to assist when the bond is terminated by death.

REFERENCE

Keddie, K. M. G. 1977. Pathological mourning after the death of a domestic pet. *British Journal of Psychiatry* 131:21–25.

5

When Pet Animals Die

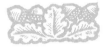

JACOB ANTELYES

VETERINARIANS often are so preoccupied with the scientific and administrative aspects of their profession they tend to lose touch with the emotional content of their work. This is particularly noticeable when the patient dies or is about to die. At such times, when the circumstances are so grave and the impact on all concerned so significant, a special sensitivity and awareness are most urgently needed. Regrettably here, more glaringly than at other times, empathy, understanding, and insight are sorely lacking.

The unfortunate fact that these qualities are also frequently wanting in human medical-surgical practice and even in psychotherapy, social work, and other helping situations does not mitigate the problem. On the contrary it only compounds and exacerbates the universal human predicament surrounding death.

Why is it so important to consider the impact on the veterinarian of the loss of his patient when the client and the animal itself are clearly under extreme stress? Because professional objectivity tends to bring about a loss of caring and this leads to two clinical sins: 1) use of jargon and 2) use of euphemisms.

If the ideal goal of veterinarians is to adapt their services to fill the client's needs, it is absolutely vital that they allow themselves to experience a patient's death personally, and then be able to express feelings about it to the owner with earnestness and sincerity. Most of us do try to do this, but we seem to accomplish it with only the greatest difficulty and awkwardness. The principal reason for our clumsy behavior is the cultural taboo, almost unassailable until recently, against open discussion of terminal illness and bereavement. Moreover it is my contention that until one has come to terms with one's own inner sentiments about death and dying, no person, including the veterinary practitioner, is capable of offering other individuals, human or animal, the total support they deserve at such a critical time. Despite the many anthropomorphic speculations permeating zoological folklore, the human being still remains the only living creature who knows with certainty about death, recognizes it as the final event in life, and feels so acutely the sense of loss it creates. Thus the fundamental conflicts in veterinarians' minds are drawn with crystal clarity. Their early education and their social and cultural backgrounds have programmed them to shun any thoughts or feelings about death, yet the clinical day is replete with fatalities, near-fatalities, and all varieties of mortal decisions.

Is it any wonder then that we so often seek to comfort bereaved owners with technical jargon? And when that fails, as it must, that we find ourselves substituting tired euphemisms for sincerity? I submit that this is true of virtually all the learned professions, but especially so in those concerned with helping others overcome the trauma of a loved one's death.

For instance, animal clinic staff members, as well as pet owners, traditionally refer to euthanasia as "putting to sleep." This is by no means the harmless and innocuous phrase it seems. At best, it is an inexpedient and unbecoming distortion, leading to ambiguity; at worst, it is an out-and-out hypocrisy, causing misunderstandings, with tragic results from time to time. Such casualties are not always psychological; they can be clinical as well. More than one pet owner has been horrified to find that his animal had been euthanized when he thought he had left it at the clinic to be "put to sleep" only during the course of an examination or treatment. Even if such misfortune is extremely rare, not even one creature should die because of communication failure between two people.

Dr. Richard C. Simmonds, a Maryland veterinarian, describes

a much more serious consequence of such misconception. A child, whose pet had recently been euthanized, was about to undergo surgery and was told that he would be "put to sleep" for the procedure. He was terror stricken, because this was exactly the term used by his parents and the veterinarian when the animal's life was ended. Fortunately, his terror was allayed when the difference between euthanasia and anesthesia was explained in clear language. But, charges Dr. Simmonds, "How many other children experience similar concerns but fail to articulate them? Obviously we need to be more careful in how we use this euphemism and try to educate our adult clients about the potential pitfalls of using this expression with their children" (Simmonds 1980).

In my own practice we try to reserve the term sleep for either natural sleep or sleep induced by anesthetics. Then there can be no possible misunderstanding about whether the patient is dead or merely resting. For intentional death we use the term euthanasia. If the client is not entirely certain of what we mean we do not hesitate to add, "This is how you give us permission to end life." Almost always we continue to offer as the reason, "to prevent further suffering."

The use of euphemisms not only causes misunderstandings and evades reality, but also erects barriers between people and increases the distance their communications must travel. These barriers and this distance are invariably emotional but are just as often physical as well. Too many professionals, including veterinarians, find themselves more comfortable "out of it," set apart from, perhaps even above, the throes of human grief. Astonishing as it may seem it is not unusual for some practitioners to assign unpleasant conversations to a staff member rather than become involved with the tragic situation themselves.

In my view it is not enough for a clinician of any calling to murmur, "I'm sorry," or, "I guess it was one of those things," and then flee from the distressing scene. The bereaved client deserves more — much more — and it is up to the practitioner to provide it.

Generally the reasons for the absence of empathic expression among professionals in our culture are quite clear. Our society places high value on what is termed the "competency cluster" of personality traits, the stereotyped male character: A strong, rational, competent individual who is tough, mature, unemotional, level-headed, and self-disciplined. On the other hand our culture considers a person with the "warmth and expressiveness cluster" of personality as second-rate, weak, frail, and less competent. We tend to stereotype the expression of feelings as a feminine trait, indicating that the person who displays this characteristic is passive, illogical, impractical, self-indulgent, and dependent.

For these reasons few professionals of any calling dare show their feelings lest they lose status. To be seen as effective in their work, practically all scientists strive to present an unfeeling exterior.

The feminist movement, over the past three decades, has made some progress in helping to alter this unreasonable social attitude. Its influence has operated mainly in the United States, however, and then principally in urban centers. The heartland remains almost as fixed as ever in its male-dominated hierarchy and its pervasive sexism.

The ultra-fearful among us may still continue to use early social conditioning as a convenient excuse for resisting change, but not, I hope, for long. Too many responsible scientists are beginning to demand an end to the substitution of euphemisms for genuine caring. The public, long weary of the frustration resulting from vain attempts to communicate with a detached, uninvolved professional, will insist on emotional support from its counselors and helpers. Eventually we will all be forced to see the unproductive and untoward sequels of our actions—the sense of alienation, of being cut off from meaningful human ties—and change.

At a 1980 symposium, "Knowlege, Education, and Human Values," sponsored by the Charles F. Kettering Foundation and the Teachers College of Columbia University, this theme was emphasized. Scientific specialization and the subsequent fragmentation of knowledge, the participants asserted, has led to a kind of tunnel vision, with each individual able to see only the narrow path to an insignificant goal. We have become disconnected from each other, our human values cheapened. We have, they maintained, "created an economic, political and educational system that values facts over curiosity, financial gains over social contributions, precision over insights," and "this method of thinking has permeated all levels of social interaction and intellectual pursuit . . ." (Kleiman 1980).

It is time for veterinarians to shift positions, to alter attitudes, to adapt to humanity. As practitioners in a helping profession, we should have matured sufficiently by now to reject as unnecessary our disjunction, our dissociation with society in general. Our status is so well developed and so firmly established that we should have absolutely no fear of increasing our contacts with human realities and responding to them.

REFERENCES

Kleiman, D. 1980. *New York Times,* June 24, section C, p. 4.
Simmonds, R. C. 1980. Put to sleep: Man vs. animal. *Journal of the American Veterinary Medical Association* 177(October 15):678.

6

Population Aspects
of Animal Mortality

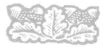

ALAN M. BECK

EACH YEAR large numbers of pet animals die from old age, disease, euthanasia, willful killing, neglect, and accident. Statistics regarding the abundance and fecundity of pet animals are inadequate so there are even poorer data regarding actual mortality. Presumably the companion animals that die of old age or disease (including animals euthanized because of terminal illness), are owned by people who experience the greatest grief upon loss. It appears, however, according to studies cited below, that the lives of most animals are terminated before old age by the intervention of humans who either actively contribute to the animal's death or neglect to provide for its basic needs, thus increasing the factors of mortality.

An active contribution to an animal's death would include willful killing or seeing to it that the animal is killed. We really don't know how often animals are directly killed by people, although cries from humane organizations suggest cruelty and neglect. Complaints about neglect may indicate that willful killing is far more common than is appreciated.

In New York City where animal ownership per capita is actually less than the national average, the American Society for Prevention of Cruelty to animals (ASPCA) investigates some 8,000 cruelty and neglect cases a year. It is quite apparent that only a small portion of such cases ever reaches the stage of being investigated.

However, the more frequently documented cases are those of animals that lose their lives because owners deliver their animal to a veterinarian or animal shelter, or deliver it to another person who subsequently gives up the animal (Beck 1974). Evidence of the active termination of life comes from many sources; at least three separate surveys have found the animal population to be declining *(DVM* 1980). As an example, from 1976 through 1977, 1978, and 1979, dog ownership went from 50 percent to 49.1 percent to 47.8 percent, and in 1979, was down to 46.5 percent. A survey from the Market Research Corporation of America (MRCA) found that dog ownership was already down to 40 percent by 1980 (R. H. Wilbur, personal communication). Cat ownership went down only 1 percent in the same 4-year period, 1976–1980. The MRCA survey found that while cat ownership per household has been holding steady in the last few years, there was, from 1972 to 1980, more than a 5 percent decline in the number of cats per household (1.9 to 1.8). Of the variety of reasons why animal ownership is decreasing the most likely is the lessening of affluence of human owners. All studies show that animal ownership is directly related to income, and per capita income may be going down (Purvis and Otto 1976).

Another source of animal mortality stems from their use in medical research; although most of these animals are specifically bred for such purposes, a small portion are former pets and strays taken from animal shelters. We have no estimates of the numbers that die, but several estimates of the total are used, representing the maximum that could be killed. The available estimates vary, but all indicate that fewer than 190,000 dogs and 69,000 cats are used each year. The majority of the nearly 1.7 million research animals used yearly are rodents, not pets (Animal Welfare Enforcement FY 1980; National Survey of Laboratory Animal Facilities and Resources 1980; USDA, Animal/Plant Health Inspection Service 1981, personal communication). Therefore the total dogs and cats used in research, not all of which die, represent less than 2 percent of the total dogs and cats that die in shelters. The animals that die in shelters were almost all former pets.

Obviously we can document much animal mortality; we know less about the reasons. In 1975 the Pet Food Institute undertook a major survey to assess some of the social and psychological attitudes about pet animal ownership. Among other questions they asked former owners the reasons for no longer owning an animal. Only 38 percent of dog owners and 24 percent of cat owners lost their animals because of illness or old age, while 35 percent of dog owners and 31 percent of cat owners gave away their animals to another person or to the ASPCA. The major reasons for giving away dogs included their being untrainable or uncontrollable, 21 percent; yards being too small, 25 percent; and pets not being permitted, 12 percent. Former cat owners reported the responsibility being too great as the single most important reason, 29 percent. Animal care costing too much as a reason for giving away a pet was indicated in less than 2 percent of the cases for both dogs and cats (Wilbur 1976), which is at odds with other observations, perhaps indicating that people are not always candid with surveyors. More than half the former owners say they will not own another pet (Wilbur 1976).

Animals are also given away because of such health reasons as bite and allergy. Animal bite is a major problem (Beck 1981a; Beck et al. 1975; Lockwood and Beck 1975), and undoubtedly many animals are released to the streets or brought to shelters and veterinarians after a bite incident. It is also not known how many people give up their animals because of allergic reactions within the family although 33 percent of 170 allergists surveyed in 1979 noted that they uniformly recommended the elimination of all pets from allergic households even if the patient did not exhibit allergic symptoms to the pet; however, they felt only about 31 percent of the patients followed their recommendations (Baker 1979).

There is also some evidence of passive termination of life. From my own studies in Baltimore I found that one-third to one-half of dog owners admitted letting their animals run free without direct supervision (Beck 1974; 1975a). There is ample evidence that free-running dogs experience a much higher mortality than responsibly owned dogs. In a national survey, 18 percent of former dog owners and 22 percent of former cat owners reported the animal was killed in an accident (Wilbur 1976).

My own studies found that most stray animals seen on streets are in fact former pets (Beck 1974; 1975b; Fox et al. 1975). Life table studies based on tooth-wear aging techniques in two different cities showed that dogs on streets experience a much shorter life expectancy than owned animals, a difference of at least 2 years

(Beck 1974). Owned dogs' average age is 4.4 years (Dorn, Terbrusch, and Hibbard 1967) compared to 2.3 years for strays (Beck 1974).

Of the lives of most companion animals that are terminated before old age by willful intervention, either actively or passively, the highest mortality appears to be in young adults. Since the population is showing only sporadic decreases, we must assume a high degree of turnover of individuals and the creation of a pet population that is unquestionably younger than would be found in a population of animals that experiences only natural sources of mortality consistent with the life span that we see in kenneled or responsibly owned individual pets.

Two major implications are in this trend. First, the grief experienced by some people associated with pet loss is not the typical response of animal owners, and second, health factors are implied by this high turnover and short life span. The fact that most people willfully separate from their pets without experiencing grief or at least *apparently* not experiencing grief may mean that the incidence of remarkable grief reactions are atypical responses not easily compared to human loss and separation. The psychological imperatives for these people may go beyond animal ownership. Owners who ask to speak with a professional social worker at the University of Pennsylvania's Veterinary Hospital at the time of the pet animal's death, reveal an indication of a more extreme grief response, and they often have concerns that go beyond their animal's death. For example an owner may say the animal's death occurred within two years of the loss of a significant person to the owner, or the owner may explain the cause of the animal's death had striking similarities to the disease causing the death of a person close to the owner.

Another hypothesis worthy of analysis is that it takes several years to form a close bond with a pet animal, but most animals are surrendered or lost within several months after coming into the home. A survey of New York State animal shelters found that of the animals received, 35.9 percent of the dogs were puppies and 45.9 percent of the cats were kittens; indicating that although juvenile pets are not the majority, they do account for a noticeable number of animal surrenders and, consequently, deaths (Argus Archives 1973).

Additional evidence that length of time together may facilitate the bond between companion animal and owner comes from some observations of the social work service at the University of Pennsylvania's Veterinary Hospital. At the time of an animal's death (from disease or euthanasia) all clients may request to speak to a social worker. Presumably people requiring such counseling have a closer bond. Owners of older animals, who almost always have had a longer association with their pets, have a much higher social service utilization rate. Only 3.4 percent of people who lose a dog under 6 years of age see the social worker; the rate goes up to 26.9 percent for dogs 6–12 years of age, and 31.3 percent for dogs 13 years and older. Less than 3 percent of cat owners use the service when the cat is less than 12 years old but the service is utilized by 40 percent of cat owners whose animal was age 13 or more. Apparently the longer time together, the more mournful the separation (J. E. Quackenbush, personal communication).

It is also tempting to speculate on the psychosocial impact of the trend toward the ownership of the larger breeds, a trend that has been noticed since the mid-1960s (Beck 1975b). The larger breeds have larger litters but shorter life spans. These factors also foster a greater population turnover, perhaps encouraging less grief but exacerbating the problems associated with a younger population with rapid population turnover. With a shift toward ownership of the smaller, longer-lived breeds there will be an increase in the number of people who noticeably grieve for their dog when it dies, but a lessening of some of the social problems associated with populations of young and ever-changing animals.

The health implications of an animal population that is young and continuously renewable are many. Many of the diseases and conditions that plague companion animals, such as canine distemper, leptospirosis, feline respiratory diseases, and canine roundworm infestations, more commonly affect younger individuals, thus further increasing turnover and mortality. This mortality affects, of course, the people who grieve for these pets. Many of these diseases have, or may have, health implications for people. Canine roundworm, for instance, is more than a veterinary problem because aberrant infection in people is being recognized as a problem, especially for children (Beck 1975b; 1979; 1981b; Schantz and Glickman 1979). In addition, rabies, the most feared zoonosis of companion animals, is more common in young animals and occurs more often in nonimmune populations. Even when rabies was a major disease in the dog population in the United States (up to 1954), about 75 percent of all exposures came from owned animals under 1 year of age. It has been shown that you can keep rabies out of the dog population if more than 70 percent of the population is immune (Beran et al. 1972; Kappus 1976). It would be very difficult to maintain this level of immunity in a population with great turnover. In fact, in parts of the world where there are rabies reservoirs in wildlife, we still see continuous rabies occurrences. I frankly believe that the major reasons we have rabies under control in the United States are first, the low level of wildlife exposure, and second, the immunization level we can maintain in the face of the rapid turnover.

One final note: the continuous loss and turnover of pet animals may foster the ambivalence our culture has exhibited toward companion animals and their owners. On the one hand pet animals are cherished companions worthy of love and protection, and on the other they are viewed as representing the more trivial part of our consumer oriented society (*Time* 1974; 1975). The grief experienced by an individual for a single pet animal is viewed as out of place when millions of pet animals are willfully killed or turned loose every year. It is difficult to seriously enforce humane laws when inhumane treatment and neglect toward animals appear to be the more common practice.

The challenge of the future is to understand the nature of the bond between animals and people and why it is for the most part such a weak bond when it is potentially so strong and important, as demonstrated by those who truly grieve for their pet animals.

REFERENCES

Argus Archives. 1973. Unwanted pets and the animal shelter. In *Argus Archives report series no. 4.* New York: Argus Archives.
Baker, E. 1979. A veterinarian looks at the animal allergy problem. *Annals of Allergy* 43:214–16.
Beck, A.M. 1974. Ecology of unwanted and uncontrolled pets. In *Proceedings of the National Conference on the Ecology of the Surplus Dog and Cat Problem,* May 21–23, Chicago, Ill.
———. 1975a. The ecology of feral and free roving dogs in Baltimore. In *The wild canids,* ed. M. W. Fox. New York: Van Nostrand Reinhold.
———. 1975b. The public health implications or urban dogs. *American Journal of Public Health* 65:1315–18.
———. 1976. Border rabies review committee. Internal report, Center for

Disease Control Investigation of US/Mexico Border Rabies. Unpublished data.

———. 1979. The impact of the canine clean-up law. *Environment* 21 (8):28–31.

———. 1981a. The epidemiology of animal bite. *Compendium on Continuing Education for the Practicing Veterinarian* 3(3) (March): 254–55; 257–58.

———. 1981b. Guidelines for planning for pets in urban areas. In *Interrelations between people and pets,* ed. B. Fogle. Springfield, Ill.: Charles C Thomas.

Beck, A.M., H. Loring, and R. Lockwood. 1975. The ecology of dog bite injury in St. Louis, Missouri. *Public Health Report* 90:262–67.

Beran, G. et al. 1972. Epidemiological and control studies on rabies in the Philippines. *Southeast Asian Journal of Tropical Medicine and Public Health* 3:433–45.

Dorn, C. R., F. G. Terbrusch, and H. H. Hibbard. 1967. *Zoographic and demographic analysis of dog and cat ownership in Alameda County, California, 1965.* Berkeley: State of California Department of Public Health.

DVM. 1980. 11(1) (January): 53.

Fox, M. W., A. M. Beck, and E. Blackman. 1975. Behavior and Ecology of a small group of urban dogs (*Canis Familaris*). *Applied Animal Ethology* 1:119–37.

Kappus, K. D. 1976. Canine rabies in the United States, 1971–1973: Study of report cases with reference to vaccination history. *American Journal of Epidemiology* 103:242–49.

Lockwood, R., and A. M. Beck. 1975. Dog bites among letter carriers in St. Louis. *Public Health Report* 90(3) (May-June):267–69.

Purvis, M. J., and D. M. Otto. 1976. Household demand for pet food and the ownership of cats and dogs: An analysis of a neglected component of U.S. food use. Staff paper, University of Minnesota, St. Paul, Department of Agriculture and Applied Economics.

Schantz, P. M., and L. T. Glickman. 1979. Canine and human toxocariasis: The public health problem and the veterinarian's role in prevention. *Journal of the American Veterinary Medical Association* 175:1270–73.

Time. 1974. The great American animal farm. 23 (December): 58–64.

Time. 1975. Forum: The great American petmania. 6 (January):58.

U.S. Department of Agriculture, Animal and Plant Health. 1980. *Animal welfare enforcement.* FY 1979. Inspection Service Report of the Secretary of Agriculture to the President of the Senate and the Speaker of the House of Representatives. Washington, D.C.: GPO.

U.S. Department of Health and Human Services. 1978. *National survey of laboratory animal facilities and resources.* NH Publ. 80–2091. Washington, D.C.: GPO.

Wilbur, R. H. 1976. Pets, pet ownership and control: Social and psychological attitudes, 1976. In *Proceedings of the National Conference on Dog and Cat Control,* February 3–5, Denver, Colo.

II

The Grieving Human Companion

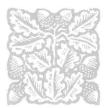

7

Grief at the Loss of a Pet

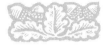

BORIS M. LEVINSON

My mind struggled with two sets of images: one a vast but amorphous panorama of nuclear war; the other of a particular, beautiful animal dying. When later on I asked myself which set of images had been the most vivid and painful, I had to confess that it had been the second, involving the dog. The anticipated death of a specific being (not even a human) had greater impact than the more total but obscure threat of extermination. The most vivid image I retain from the experience is that of the dog, a large and formerly spirited creature, lying still on the floor of the veterinary hospital. (Lifton 1979, 367)

WITH THE DYNAMIC CHANGES occurring in American life (the decrease in size of families and the virtual disappearance of extended families), animal companions are beginning to play greater roles in people's lives. The death of a pet may be a traumatic, almost catastrophic event in the life of the owner, especially when the owner has not been able to trust other humans and has turned to a pet for unconditional love and support. Since they belong to one of the social species, the animals most often made into pets can both acknowledge affection and give it in return (Levinson 1972a; 1980b).

Grieving is a complex emotional experience. The nature of the mourning reaction will depend upon what the pet has meant to its owner or owners. Was the animal regarded as a companion, a toy, a protector, a confidante, a child? In each case the human reaction to the loss of the animal would be different, just as it is when a beloved person dies. It will also depend on the age and stage of development of the mourner, since adults and children react in distinctive ways (Peterson and McCabe 1977–1978). The death of an animal companion may also bring about a shifting in the roles of the various family members and a change in their interaction with each other, necessitating a readjustment in the way the family functions. The grief that is expressed for a pet sometimes serves a dual purpose. Some people, especially children, find it difficult to accept the reality of the death of a loved human, whether parent, sibling, spouse, or child, and therefore cannot fully mourn for the lost person. They can, however, shed tears for a lesser love object, such as a dog or cat. By grieving for the pet they evoke memories of the loved person who has been lost and thus can gradually accept, mourn, and assimilate the death that previously they could only deny.

A recent widow, who had been quite controlled and cried little at her husband's death, was stricken soon afterward by the death of a much-loved cat. Her grief seemed inconsolable and her tears unquenchable. She kept lamenting: "But I took such good care of him." The question that occurs immediately is: about whom was this widow weeping – her cat or her husband? (Antelyes, personal communication, 1972)

Such displaced mourning, incidentally, occurs not only through pets but through other important losses as well (loss of one's home or job, for example) (Fried 1963).

Depending on the circumstances of the animals' death, the mourning process will show different features in the human survivors. When death occurs from natural causes, the owners experience a variety of feelings. There is shock, especially if the death had not been anticipated and prepared for. Although adults know that animals such as dogs and cats do not live as long as humans, children may not know this and need to be accustomed to this idea while the animal is still well. Adults, too, need to learn to recognize the signs of old age in a companion animal.

When the pet is ill, both adults and children have to be able to experience anticipatory grief so that they can make psychological preparations for its death, talking about it as a possibility and even a probability within a given length of time. Many children appear to be unconcerned about the pet's illness and act as though it did not exist, believing that if one doesn't talk about illness it will go away. They must be helped to recognize that this magical way of dealing with an unacceptable reality will not prevent the feared event (Levinson 1972b; 1978; 1980a; Montefiore et al. 1973). At the point when the animal dies, anger, protest, and guilt often surface. Why this pet and not someone else's? Why at this age, when many pets live longer? Why at such an inopportune time? Why didn't the veterinarian give the animal better or different care? Children may blame their parents for having been stingy and not having done enough to save the animal. They may also blame themselves for having neglected the pet, not having played enough with it, brushed it enough, taken it out for airings often enough or at the right time. Sometimes children interpret the death of the pet as punishment for their misdeeds. They may then fear that future misdeeds will result in their own deaths (Levinson 1972a).

Both adults and children may idealize their dead pet, remembering only the pleasant times and forgetting the unpleasant details of living with the animal—the obligation to walk it no matter how inconvenient, the pet's occasional "accidents" and destruction of valued property. The reexperiencing of the good times is a healing experience, especially for children who have been given some memento of their pet.

It is a temptation for some parents not to tell their children that the beloved pet has died. Fearing the pain that the children will experience if they are told the truth, or being unwilling themselves to acknowledge the loss and thus experience the pain it brings, they fabricate stories about the animal's disappearance from the scene, hoping that the children will eventually forget they ever had a pet. Thus they tell the children that the animal has been taken on a trip or is visiting friends in the country and won't return for some time. Eventually the children learn the "truth" or some fantasied interpretation supplied by neighbors and friends, and this may seriously shake their confidence in their parents' trustworthiness and prevent their believing what is told to them about anything. This is much more harmful to children than the pain they will experience over the death of their loved animal. Children are not as fragile as most of us assume. Telling them the truth in a gentle, sensitive fashion not only permits them to trust and rely on the strength displayed by their parents under this bereavement, but also serves as a kind of inoculation for the greater pain of loss they may experience in the future at the death of parents, close relatives, and intimate friends. By giving children an opportunity to experience and express their feelings about the pet's death and to ask questions about it, we are also helping them to come to terms with their own and everyone else's mortality. "Will this happen to you, too?" a child may ask. "Will it happen to me?" "Why?" "Where did he go?" "Will we ever see him again?" "Does an animal have a soul?" Parents must answer in terms of their own beliefs, always bearing in mind that children will create their own fantasies to explain what has happened, coming up with an explanation which may have little to do with reality or what the parents have told them, but which makes sense to them at that point in their development.

Parents may want to tell a child that the pet continues to live with the family through the good memories they have of him or her and the love that was shared. They may want to point out that the pet is now helping other things grow, becoming part of the trees and grass as it lies in the ground. Mementos of the animal—pictures, a leash, a feeding cup—may also be described as ways in which the animal continues to be part of the family. The children should be encouraged to express feelings, and no attempt should be made to talk them out of them, no matter how sad or angry they may be.

When pet owners are faced with a terminally ill and suffering animal, they must make the difficult and painful decision as to whether to euthanize it. On the one hand it is cruel to permit a loved animal to suffer needlessly and it can even be considered an owner's responsibility to provide his pet a quick and painless death. To keep the animal alive because we can't bear the pain of parting is selfish. Moreover, it is assumed, everything possible has been done to heal the animal, even perhaps to the point of spending more money than is readily available. In some cases one veterinarian after another has been consulted and all the recommended surgical procedures have been tried, to no avail. Now, then, both for the family's benefit and the animal's, euthanasia should be performed. Yet the pet has become a member of the family, and the decision to put it to death feels somewhat like telling one's grandmother that she has outlived her usefulness and the investment one is willing to make in her, and that it is time for her to die.

The guilt this engenders may be deepened if we have a relative who is in the terminal stages of an illness and is taking time about dying. We may wish we could do away with this person the way we can do away with our animal companion, feeling appalled at such a wish but also at our anger that such an option is not available for humans. Occasionally the pet will be the stand-in for such anger, just as it can be for grief.

A man who had been weighed down for many years by the prolonged illness of his wife discovered after her death that his cat was losing its eyesight, although otherwise it was fit. The love he had heretofore felt for the cat became sudden hatred, expressed in the order to his veterinarian, "I want you to kill my cat" (Levinson 1972b).

Some animal lovers whose own deaths appear imminent or who are contemplating suicide have their pets euthanized in the mistaken belief that no one will be available to care for the animal after the owner is gone. When these individuals recover, as they sometimes do, they may go into a depression upon realizing the loss they have inflicted on themselves. They would have done better to have made provisions for their pet in the event of their own death.

The veterinarian who is called upon to perform the euthanasia also is faced with difficult decisions. Is the euthanasia justified in terms of the animal's condition? Should the veterinarian push for euthanasia when s/he knows that cure of a severe illness, such as cancer, is improbable, and that both pet and family are suffering from the animal's condition? How does the veterinarian, especially if a neophyte, feel about performing the euthanasia?

If the veterinarian is reluctant to accede to the family's request to euthanize an animal, s/he can take various steps: s/he can turn the pet over to a humane society which may arrange for its adoption; s/he can refuse to euthanize the pet of a client s/he does not know personally until s/he has had a chance to check with friends and relatives to determine if the owner is making the request under the impact of a personal emotional stress rather than the animal's own condition; s/he can counsel the client and even direct her or him to appropriate mental health practitioners for help in clarifying the motives for requesting euthanasia.

When it is the veterinarian rather than the family who is convinced that euthanasia is advisable, the former should always place the burden of decision on the family, discussing the pros and cons, giving a full picture of the animal's condition and prognosis, and avoiding being placed in a position where s/he can later be blamed for the pet's "untimely" death (Levinson 1972b).

Once the euthanasia has been performed, the veterinarian must be able to handle the family's bereavement, especially in those cases referred to earlier where grief over the animal's death is in part a displacement from the grief over a loved person's death which has been kept out of awareness up to that point.

When a pet dies in an accident, no one is prepared for the loss. There may be guilt that the animal was not sufficiently protected, that it was allowed to run off the leash and dash into the street where it was hit by a car. There may also be anger at the pet for having been disobedient and impulsive, thus bringing about its own death.

Children are especially prone to such feelings, since they are both dependent on adult protection and apt to disobey safety rules on impulse. Children may, therefore, violently deny the fact of the pet's death, insisting, "It isn't true!" They may close their ears to words of comfort or refuse to share feelings of guilt and sorrow, instead expressing these through misbehavior which leads to punishment. They may blame their parents or even themselves for not preventing the accident, even though neither they nor their parents were present at the time it occurred.

Children may identify with the pet to such an extent that they develop fears, have nightmares and nameless terrors, expecting that they will meet the same fate as their pet and convinced that the parents cannot be counted on to protect them as they could not be counted on to protect the animal. Children may be afraid to risk new attachments, whether to animals or people, leading them to experience depressive reactions in adulthood.

When a pet disappears, either because it has run away, gotten separated from its master while being walked and not been found, or been abducted, the uncertainty as to its fate is harder for the owners to bear than knowing that the pet is dead. The owners feel deserted and abandoned by their animal companion, and also anguished at imagining how abandoned by them the animal must feel.

This was vividly illustrated by the reactions of a group of 9- to 12-year-old boys in a residential treatment center when the dog who had been so important to them got lost after chasing a car full of children going to town. They organized search parties and devised various schemes to get the animal back. Their fears, guilt, and remorse were plain. "The night is coming on and he will be terribly lonely." "Right out there in the dark forest a witch will get him." "He is scared of the giants; they'll eat him up." "Maybe he will drown himself because he is so unhappy." "Maybe he just ran away 'cause you weren't nice to him." "Maybe we didn't give him enough food." "Maybe he just stopped loving us." Most poignant was the promise of a boy who couldn't care about a soul in the world, "Tell God I'm never, never gonna be nasty if he sends Levinson back." (Levinson 1969, 109–10)

This identification with an animal's sense of terror and pain at being deprived of the master on whom it is dependent for its life has led some wealthy people to leave the bulk of their estate to their pets rather than to relatives.

Not knowing whether the loss is temporary or permanent, the owners keep their hopes alive and cannot begin the mourning process. They hang onto their pet's dish and leash, leave its pillow and blanket in its usual spot, thus facing a daily reminder of their loss along with the denial of the reality of the loss. One couple who lost their poodle offered a $1,000 reward for his return, the wife explaining that the dog had become so much a member of the family that "it's ruined my life, losing him."

The disappearance of a pet may reinforce in both child and

adult feelings that the world is not a safe place, that one's security can abruptly be destroyed. It plays into the child's deepest fears that s/he will be deprived of the protection and nurturance of her or his parents without which s/he cannot survive. To get lost, to be left behind, to be carried off are fears that never entirely leave us, no matter how old we get. As parents, we have the same fears where our children are concerned. A lost or stolen pet touches many deep feelings of both children and adults while preventing relief from being achieved through the mourning process. Eventually, of course, there is a presumption of death or at least of permanent loss.

As in the case of the death of a loved human, burial rites can serve to initiate the process of mourning. For children this is particularly important.

Children who have described the burial of their pets, while revealing a strong element of drama, imitation, and play in the activity, also reveal much genuine grief and tenderness and a "desire that the dead pet shall be gently cared for and respect shown to her memory. Flowers are placed on the grave, not only at the time of the funeral but the successive seasons." (Hall and Browne 1904, 25)

An 18-year-old student, in a group asked to remember any rituals associated with death in their childhood, reported: "I remember the death of my budgerigar. We made a special wooden coffin, placed him tenderly on cotton wool, and had a procession down the garden with a cross." (Mitchell 1967)

An adult man looked back on the burial of his dog as follows:

I wonder if any canine requiem could ever compare to Sandy's. Three youthful self-ordained priests presided, one eulogized. His cardboard casket was covered with a black pall, lowered away to an off-key Gregorian chant. Mother made the priestly vestments, and we served lots of his favorite Necco wafers, white ones, to all the Protestant kids who came to gawk. We buried him in ground blessed with our own homemade holy water. Then we rolled a huge rock over his grave.

In retrospect, it all sounds so cute and boyish. At the time it was not. It was sad and upsetting, somewhat frightening. I felt uneasy digging a grave, lifting my dead dog, throwing dirt over him, all the while wondering if there might be a dog heaven. My teacher, Sister Mary, said there well could be. I think I prayed for Sandy every time we walked along the path where we laid him in case there was a purgatory for dogs, too. (Kavanaugh 1972, 22)

Children's attempts at mastering the loss by actively acknowledging it through a ritual of farewell are sometimes misunderstood by well-meaning adults who attempt to prevent the activity and thus possibly leave the child feeling helpless and overwhelmed.

He (Roscoe), too, was discouraged from open expression of concern. Roscoe's ritualistic behavior around, and preoccupation with, the burying of dead animals in a backyard graveside was looked upon as "morbid" by professionals and teachers. They recommended aversive training as a remedy. The behavior was not seen as a piece of anticipatory mourning, nor understood as an effort at active mastery. Its healthful and adaptive functions were overriden by cultural squeamishness and clinical adherence to notions of psychopathology. (Berman 1973, 103)

Adults, too, are faced with a decision about disposing of the body of a dead pet. Most of the time the choice is made between leaving the task up to the veterinarian or arranging for private cremation or burial. Inhabitants of rural areas who have their own land available may choose to bury their animal on home ground. In large cities it is usually contrary to the health code to bury an animal on one's own or public property within city limits. Some cities have animal cemeteries on their outskirts or animal crematoria.

Pet funerals have become quite common among owners who find it crude and heartless to allow pickup of their dead pet's body by the town garbage truck. Few funerals, however, are as lavish as that given to the pet terrier of a Georgian man, which included the reading of scripture over an embalmed body, five dozen rosebuds, four pallbearers, and a funeral procession of several cars for a total cost of $1,000. The owner, denying that his actions were extravagant, asked reporters, "Who else in the world has found a million dollars worth of happiness for $1,000?" (Rice 1968, 133)

The Bonheur Memorial Park Cemetery in Elkridge, Md. calling itself the only pet cemetery in the world where humans could be buried next to their pets, reported last November that it would expand. It asked the Howard County Board of Appeals for a zoning variance to develop an economy cemetery for the pets of "blue-collar workers earning $10,000 to $12,000 a year."

A five-acre cemetery two miles from the existing one has been approved, and the new burial ground will open this week, reports the owner, William Green. It is for pets only.

"We've got about 17, 18 dogs to go in there so far," he says. "We've got them in refrigeration."

Whereas pet burials in the main cemetery can range in cost to $1,700 (with velvet-lined mahogany coffin and bronze grave marker), those in the economy cemetery will be $85 to $125 (with plywood coffin and tin marker). All pet coffins are enclosed in a concrete vault before burial, Mr. Green stresses.

"I'm a very strong believer in that," he says. "You got a lot of places that say, 'We've got a combination casket-vault here; you don't need a vault with it.' Well, you know, you wouldn't bury your wife without a vault, so you're not going to bury your pet without one." (New York Times 1981)

Sometimes mourning for a pet reaches a pathological degree, whether by its intensity or excessive duration. The connection between severe depression in some people and the prior loss of a pet has not, for the most part, been recognized by mental health professionals who have thought that the role of an animal companion in a person's emotional economy is insufficiently important to serve as a cause for an emotional disorder.

However, other clinicians have been aware that a severe reaction to the death of a pet may occur if the person has lacked emotional fulfillment and closeness to other people. Those who for one reason or another have been shunned by society or avoided human attachments out of fear or distrust may have displaced their capacity for forming an affectional bond to an animal, which is seen as nonjudgmental, undemanding, and intensely loyal (Keddie 1977; Rynearson 1978). In such people, the death of a pet may so frustrate the need for closeness and attachment that the response is a tragic one. One such case was that of a lonely separated woman whose only remaining source of love was her affectionate dog, and who "literally lost her reason when, on returning home, she found her pet gone. She wandered, inconsolable, looking for her pet until she collapsed." (Arsenian 1973, 53)

Psychiatrist E. K. Rynearson (1978) hypothesizes that some people who have received inadequate parenting can feel safe only with animals as attachment figures. This psychiatrist describes three cases of intense, prolonged mourning following the death of a pet. In one case a woman who had become a recluse because of selfconsciousness over her bulging eyes, became unable to separate from the family dog, so that he slept with her at night and was never out of her sight until he died. In another case, a woman whose husband had suddenly died "saw" in her husband's coffin not his body but that of her childhood pet cat which her mother had murdered in a fit of rage. In a third case, a woman killed herself and her dog following a bitter quarrel over the "custody" of the dog to which both mother and daughter were pathologically attached as a means of remaining symbiotically intertwined with each other. Other suicides on the death of a pet have also been recorded (Levinson 1972a).

Though not producing such dire consequences, perpetual bereavement is also pathological and indicative of the use of the animal to deal with some inner conflict. Mrs. R, for example, has been in perpetual mourning since the death of her Yorkshire terrier five years ago. The dog's picture is draped in black. Pictures throughout her apartment depict scenes from the life of the departed dog. A separate room is consecrated to the dog's belongings: his dish, leash, etc. Mrs. R is depressed and her constant talk is about her dog. It would seem that Mrs. R is and was only an unimportant extension of the more important part of herself — the dog — which is gone forever.

Sometimes the death of an animal companion does not seem to trouble its owner. Mr. C, a man of 70, had a Shetland sheepdog, which had been a constant companion for 10 years until it was killed in an auto accident. Mr. C did not seem to react to the loss of his companion, and went about his business as if nothing had happened. He was the only survivor in his family of a Nazi extermination camp where his wife and four children had perished. Mr. C never had a chance to resolve his grief and therefore had to erect a defense against further loving. Since the concentration camp experience he had decided, on an unconscious level, never to become emotionally attached to another person or animal. To love and lose again would mean to him a repetition of his entire tragic past.

A child I am currently treating in psychotherapy, Tony, had a dog and cat, his most cherished possessions, which perished in a fire. This bereavement has never been resolved, and it has become most difficult to treat the child's underlying psychological problems. Tony firmly believes he is "bad." If this were not so why would he have been punished by having his two pets taken away from him? Any attempt to convince him he is not bad and deserving of dire punishment leads him to turn against the therapist and try to provoke a situation where restraining him is necessary. As a result he is not likeable nor liked. In this child's mind, he is "proving" he is as bad as he thinks he is.

Should you replace your old friend when it dies? That depends. Some owners may feel their pet represents something irreplaceable in their lives, a link to the past for which there is no substitute. This sense of continuity was well expressed by Charles Dickens in *David Copperfield* when Dora refuses another dog to replace her little Jip:

> I couldn't be friends with any other . . . because he wouldn't have known me before I was married, and wouldn't have barked at Doady when he first came to the house. . . . He has known me in all that has happened to me. . . . (Papashvilly 1954, 144).

Sometimes adults and children alike feel guilty over the real or imagined neglect of their beloved pet in life, so that when the pet dies they feel they would be betraying him twice by acquiring a replacement. Out of such a feeling of guilt a child may reject a new pet brought into the household by the parents, and may even kill it.

We have also seen people who, when their pet dies, swear never to get another one because bereavement is so painful they are afraid to love again. However, most pet owners decide to replace a dead animal companion after a period of mourning has taken place. Children who want an immediate substitute for their lost pets should be allowed to grieve for a while so that they learn that friendships, even those with animals, cannot easily be replaced. When a new pet is acquired, it should not be looked upon as a replacement for the old one, which is something it cannot be. It is a companion in its own right and must be accepted for what it is, which does not, of course, prevent children from thinking now and then about their old friends. Children also learn as they come to love the replacement "that life must go on." (Levinson 1980a, 72) In some situations, for example, when a child is in the family and a sick pet is going to die, it may be advisable to bring in a younger pet before that happens. The child can in this way become accustomed to the new pet, come to like it, and consider it a friend. Thus when the old animal dies the child will have the new one for comfort. This may be better than replacing a pet after it dies.

To sum up, human grief over the death of an animal companion is a very real and ubiquitous phenomenon. Moreover, as a demonstration of the human capacity to love and form attachments, it is a hopeful sign in an age where feelings of alienation have reached epidemic proportions.

REFERENCES

Arsenian, J. 1973. Situational factors contributing to mental illness in the elderly. In *Death anxiety,* ed. H. W. Montefiore et al. New York: MSS Information Corporation.
Berman, E. 1973. *Scapegoat.* Ann Arbor: University of Michigan Press.
Fried, M. 1963. Grieving for a lost home. In *The urban condition,* ed. L. Duhl. New York: Basic Books.
Hall, S. G., and C. E. Browne. 1904. The cat and the child. *Pedagogical Seminary* 11:3–29.
Kavanaugh, R. E. 1972. *Facing death.* Los Angeles: Nash.
Keddie, K. M. G. 1977. Pathological mourning after the death of a domestic pet. *British Journal of Psychiatry* 131:21–25.
Levinson, B. M. 1969. *Pet-oriented child psychotherapy.* Springfield, Ill.: Charles C Thomas.
_____. 1972a. *Pets and human development.* Springfield, Ill.: Charles C Thomas.
_____. 1972b. Man and his feline pet. *Modern Veterinary Practice* 53:35–39.
_____. 1978. Pets and personality development. *Psychological Reports* 42:1031–38.
_____. 1980a. The child and his pet: A world of non-verbal communication. In *Ethology and non-verbal communication in mental health,* ed. S. A. Corson and E. O'Leary Corson. London: Pergamon.
_____. 1980b. Acute grief in animals. Paper presented at the Foundation of Thanatology symposium, Acute Grief, New York, N.Y. (November).
Lifton, R. J. 1979. *The broken connection.* New York: Simon and Schuster.
Mitchell, M. 1967. *The child's attitude to death.* New York: Schocken.
Montefiore, H. W. et al., eds. 1973. *Death anxiety.* New York: MSS Information Corporation.

New York Times. 1981. Undertaker for pets. March 3, p. 41.

Papashvilly, H. G., and H. Papashvilly. 1954. *Dogs and people.* Philadelphia: Lippincott.

Peterson, M. C. L., and A. McCabe. 1977–1978. Children talk about death. *Omega* 8:305–18.

Rice, B. 1968. *The other end of the leash.* Boston: Little, Brown.

Rynearson, E. K. 1978. Humans and pets and attachment. *British Journal of Psychiatry* 133:550–55.

Wilbur, R. H. 1976. Pets, pet ownership and control: Social and psychological attitudes. In *Proceedings of the National Conference on Dog and Cat Control,* February 3–4, 1976, Denver, Colo.

8

Psychosocial Aspects
of Bereavement

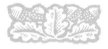

HERBERT A. NIEBURG

MANY PROFESSIONALS in the field of bereavement and grief therapy enter by a serendipitous route. Some years ago, I began to deal with cancer patients and was surprised to find that when dying people began to pick out significant others with whom they wanted to spend the last bit of quality time, very often the significant other they chose was their pet. Obviously this does not go down well with a spouse or the children or the grandchildren. "I always said your dog was more important than I am," is a frequently heard lament. And in some cases that is a very valid perception. So I became involved in the area of pet-related grief while observing this phenomenon and then proceeded with research into this area (Nieburg and Fischer 1982).

Following the publication of an article about research related to pet loss being done at the Animal Medical Center in New York City, I received a letter, which read in part:

I am writing in reference to a recent article in the *New York Times* regarding the death of a pet. Three years ago, I lost a dog that had been with me for 18 years. I was seven years old when he came to me and I was deeply attached to him. I still have a great deal of trouble dealing with his death and it is not an easy subject to discuss. I never really realized that other adults might also have trouble coming to terms with this problem. Would it be possible for you to send me further information on your studies? I would be very grateful.

I think the word *grateful* is important. Until very recently, people who sustained pet-related loss had no one to talk with about it. If they were lucky, their veterinarian was a compassionate, caring human being who could empathize and help. However, very frequently, people either did not know such a person or did not avail themselves of that kind of help. Hence they went through the loss alone and never really confronted it.

In a letter, a 10-year-old boy wrote about his dog, a pet that was about to be euthanized because of inoperable cancer that was causing pain—pain that could not be palliated or alleviated in any manner:

Why? It's all stupid Dr. Smith's fault. He could have found it sooner. Then we could operate on her leg or amputate it and she would be with us for two more years. Oh, my darling girl, my beautiful Mumu. Why did it have to be her? It's like a nightmare. It's too sad for me, I can't stand it. I wish I believed in God, then I wouldn't be sad right now because I would believe that she would get better. It's too hard for me. She'll never know what I'll look like with my teeth all fixed and my braces off. Only three days. I can't stand it. I wish I could commit suicide. Then it would solve my problem about feeling sad. But you would be even sadder, Mother. It's too hard for me. Oh, my pretty girl. She looks so healthy. Cancer. You told me just straight out. It's too sad for me. Couldn't you be more gentle? I feel angry and mad and sad all together. I don't know what mood I'm in. Just when everything is so good. I'm home from camp and we have a new tennis court, and we're going to the Bahamas. We should cancel our trip. How can we enjoy ourselves? I wish it weren't happening. Why Jody? I'm going to feel so sad when I come home from school and she isn't there to greet me. Oh, my lovey! I always liked to lie down with her when I finished playing. I don't want her to go away from me. I like to fluff her ears. Remember how she chased the diaper? My stomach hurts. I'll always remember her. There'll never be a dog as wonderful as my lovely Jody. I'll never love another dog as much. I wish a doctor would discover a cure for cancer tomorrow; then we could save her. How do you catch it? Can I get it from her? How does it start? I can't believe it's happening. Only three days . . . I want to spend as much time with her as I can. I've been away from her for seven weeks, and now only three days. She smells so good after a bath. Will you give her a bath before she goes to Dr. Smith? Can we give the new dog a bath so she smells good? I wish she would die like [and he describes his great-grandfather who died in his sleep]. This is more like killing her. I don't want her to have terrible pain. We'll all be so sad to bring her in. Papa likes to give her cheese and Meem likes to feed her chicken broth. They'll be so sad because they love my Mumu. How can this be happening? I want to teach the new dog to jump for a biscuit and all the tricks that Jody knows but not any new ones. I want a new dog before school starts. Can we get one soon? I want it to come to the door. I want it to come when I get home from school. I don't want to see an empty cubby when I come home. Can the new dog sleep in my room? I'll never be able to fall asleep. I'm too sad. I feel happy about getting a new dog, but that's mean to my Mumu.

I wish every person were able to verbalize his feelings in the way that this young boy did. The interesting thing about the letter is that it demonstrates all the emotions experienced in bereavement over the loss of a significant human: from the denial to the anger, to the isolation, to the replacement, to the identification, to the bargaining.

People become responsible pet owners for many reasons. Certain of these are practical: the barn cat, the cat in the grocery store, the guide dog, the watchdog. Other reasons have emotional bases. We know about love, companionship, and esteem needs ("my dog is bigger than your dog"; "How many ribbons do you have?"). Security is another common reason for owning pets.

Some security needs pets fulfill are definitely justified; however, I am not sure that the methods by which we turn animals into security dogs are justified. For example more and more childless couples are choosing animals as surrogate children. People are electing not to enter into the legal contract of marriage or they are deciding not to have children. Frequently we see individuals who are coping with pet loss and who essentially have identified the pet as a child. We know that pets share complementary drives and responses. In talking about human/pet attachments, we are talking about a complementary system. Before too long the family therapists who are describing the systems theory of family therapy will begin to take a look at the human/pet bond as being one of those systems. We know that people are compulsive caregivers. Why do people attach so strongly to pets in certain situations?

Areas of concern in pet loss are varied. What are some of the things that a bereavement or grief therapist is involved in when dealing with pet loss? Certainly *sudden death*. Sudden death presents a catastrophic, acute problem and requires intervention. I work very closely with veterinarians and psychotherapists. One of the key pieces of advice I offer, certainly in terms of what one does when pets die suddenly, is that sometimes you do nothing. You try to make some sort of arrangement so that people can think through what they would like to do. Sudden death can be accidental, purposeful, preventable, or negligent. Obviously we all look with dismay when a pet dies or is seriously injured because of a factor clearly recognizable as negligence on the pet owner's part. This may precipitate profound reactions.

I have discussed with veterinarians the phenomenon of people regretting what they have done and the decisions they have made under stressful conditions. We should endeavor to give people the option of waiting, whether this means going to the cold room with the pet to think about what's happening, or whatever other action is appropriate.

Where there is a chronic illness that will lead to death, we need to be concerned about preparation. People need to be told what is wrong with their pets. They need to be told diagnoses and prognoses. But more important, they need to be told in terms they will understand. It is one thing to come home and say, "My dog has a tumor and the doctor said he's going to die." It is another thing to know what the options are in terms of the kind of malignancy and perhaps what some of the statistics are so that one can deal with it psychologically.

We are aware that denial is probably the major defense mechanism observed in most people. We know the treatment of denial in many cases is to maintain the denial until the person is ready to give it up. If denial is destroyed too precipitously or prematurely, we run the risk of arousing other problems or removing a defense mechanism that is very valuable. All defense mechanisms are present for a reason and not just by coincidence.

Acceptance of a loss can be difficult. Many people do accept their pet's loss. Animal funeral directors and the International Association of Pet Cemeteries observe that acceptance is frequently manifested when people finally know what they want to do with the pet and how they can best remember that pet. At this point, a decision can be made and an action taken.

In my opinion two types of losses are experienced: Type I is voluntary, usually nondeath related, and in a situation where we have some choice. With the seriously ill pet the question of initiating chemotherapy exists or, do we need to do nothing and euthanize the animal? Type II losses are those in which we do not have a choice. A dog has bitten three people and the judge orders the animal destroyed or sent to a farm where it can roam freely. (I am not sure about the wisdom of allowing the dog to go unrestrained if it has already bitten three people, but this does happen.) This decision is one in which we have no choice. Type II loss also may involve stolen pets. Runaway pets and stolen pets evoke similar reactions — at least in my clinical experience. There is the problem of imagining what is happening to the pet. Where is it? Is it being treated humanely?

Grief is an alteration in mood and affect consisting of sadness appropriate to the real loss. This, in technical language, is saying that loss is inevitable, grieving is acceptable, and any response that we have to a loss is going to result in some sort of a grief reaction. Coping with grief is experimenting with and accepting the reality of the loss; working through memories and affect; gaining new attachments and object relationships. To counsel people in all types of losses we must identify what the problems are, what they are telling themselves about the problems, and suggest practical, how-to-do-it approaches in terms of dealing with these problems.

Normal grief is not a disorder, not a neurosis. One of the most important things counselors should do is let people know it is all right to grieve for pets, no matter what kind of creature they have chosen as their pet. Frequently, comments of, "Well, it's only a dog, it's only a pet," are heard. Yet it should be recognized that for some people pets are the real people they have chosen to deal with in their lives.

REFERENCE

Nieburg, H. A., and A. Fischer. 1982. *Pet loss: a thoughtful guide for adults.* New York: Harper and Row.

9

Relief and Prevention of Grief

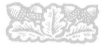

LEO K. BUSTAD, LINDA M. HINES

THE NEWSPAPER HEADLINE read, WITHOUT SPARKY, MISTRESS DIES. The article reported the death of a 77-year-old woman who had died of what her friends insisted was a "broken heart." Her life had been shattered when housing officials enforced no-pet regulations. The woman lived in a senior housing project, and the officials required her to either find another place to live or give up her dog. She had little income and no other place to go so she took the dog to the local humane society. According to her friends, giving up the dog broke her spirit and snuffed out her will to live. She stopped taking daily walks, refused to bathe, and almost stopped eating.

Much is implied in this story as to the importance of the bond between people and animals. Sparky was a source of unconditional love and affection for this woman. He gave her something to live for, ordered her life, and encouraged exercise and social contact. The severance of this bond resulted in great stress and intense grief, both of which contributed to her death.

However, the grief manifested following the loss of a companion animal need not be as destructive as that in this illustration. If managed effectively and if the loss is from natural causes, the grief can be a growing experience that strengthens the human/companion animal bond. This was well stated in a letter from an 86-year-old friend:

It was a sad day for me when Topsy, too, had to leave me. She had lived a long and happy life, for twelve years in a dog's life is calculated to be the same as over 80 in a human's. She had enriched the lives of all who knew and loved her and had given back that love in double portion! What the world would have missed if mother and I hadn't been guided that day to take an unfamiliar road back home, and her little life had been snuffed out because she was a female and nobody wanted her. How I missed her for a long, long time! And my eyes would often fill with tears when I would come home from town and there was no little dog to come bounding to the door with her "welcome home" bark. Now many years later, I count among those blessings, as one of God's sweetest gifts to me, the love of a little dog!

Health professionals, especially veterinarians, have a unique opportunity and obligation to maximize the positive experiences of such people as Topsy's owner while, it is to be hoped, eliminating the traumas faced by persons such as Sparky's owner (Bustad 1980). How can this awesome task be accomplished? First we must understand and accept grief as a legitimate subject of inquiry affecting both animals and people. Animals can teach us much about the causes, processes, and manifestations of grief (and joy, as well).

Some animals, like people, grieve. Lorenz (1952) observed this in a greylag goose, which had lost a mate. The goose was anxious and restless, flying ever-greater distances in search of the mate, visiting places where the mate might have been found, incessantly calling with a long distance call.

Bowlby (1961) described bereavements in jackdaws, geese, domestic dogs, orangutans, and chimpanzees. Each species sought to recover a lost loved object and did all in its power to achieve this. Frequent hostility, withdrawal, rejection of a potential new object, apathy, and restlessness figured in the animals' responses to their losses.

Three much-celebrated dogs manifested at least some of the symptoms of the illness we call grief. Old Shep was owned by an elderly sheepherder near Fort Benton, Montana. The sheepherder died and the dog accompanied the casket to the railroad station at Fort Benton, where it was placed on a railroad car, never, of course, to return. Old Shep established residence at the railroad yards and met every train that came into Fort Benton for more than 5 years. On 12 January 1942 he slipped, fell under the wheels of an approaching train, and was killed. A monument was erected in Old Shep's honor.

The second dog was Corky, a fox terrier, whose mistress (14-year-old Angelene) died tragically in a fire at her school. Corky ran away from his home three times and was found sitting in front of the fire-scarred building. Angelene's mother confined Corky to their home. The dog proceeded to crawl under the child's bed, did not appear for four days, and refused food. Finally, the dog began to eat again and eventually recovered (Parkes 1974).

The third dog, Hachi, is the most celebrated dog in Japan. A Tokyo University professor obtained Hachi when he was a pup. Before long, the dog began accompanying the professor to the railroad station in the morning and awaiting his return there in the evening. Together, they would walk home. Two years later, the professor died, but the dog still came to the railroad station each day, even though the family had moved to another part of Tokyo. Hachi continued to make his daily sojourns to the station until he died ten years later. A memorial statue established at the railroad station for Hachi was melted down during World War II. But following the war a new one was erected (Parkes 1974).

Quite a number of animals other than dogs manifest unusual behavior following the loss of a close associate, whether it is a person or another animal. Such animals include birds, sheep, goats, and especially nonhuman primates.

Marais (1939), in a fascinating book about his adventures following a troop of baboons in South Africa, described a memorable incident when the troop began losing a number of infants one night. He had constructed temporary quarters for himself near the baboons' sleeping quarters, a place where he was never allowed at night by the animals. One night he was awakened by the distraught leaders of the baboon troop. He accompanied them to the sleeping quarters but detected only strange behavior. Early the next morning he was awakened by "the sound of lamentation," and he then discovered a number of infants had died during the night. According to Marais:

What we heard was the terrible blood-freezing cry of woe from the baboons — persistent and heart-rending. It is almost impossible to exaggerate the effect of this sound on the human being. On most occasions it sounded, to our ears, more moving than even the cry of mourning of human beings, just because the lamentation of the baboons is wordless. It is a purely emotional sound more or less similar to the inarticulate groaning and sighing by which the deepest anguish of the human heart finds speechless expression.

Marais then described how one of the grieving young mothers followed him, emitting begging sounds:

She wanted exactly what the seven large males, who had visited us so unexpectedly the previous evening, had wanted—our help to ward off approaching death from the infants—that approaching death of which in all probability they had become aware the previous evening. And the mother wanted from us the revival of her child. She wanted to have changed that huge and remorseless condition which in her environment she had learnt to know as death.

Pollock (1961) related an observation concerning the death of a large infant in a troop of baboons. The mother had left the infant, but the largest male of the troop refused to leave it and began a screaming and barking that ceased only when the mother returned to retrieve her baby. This scene was repeated several times before they reached their sleeping trees. It was probably difficult for the mother to carry the baby, for she had to walk and run on three legs while holding the dead baby. This would be uncommon for baboons since a baby of such size usually jumps on the mother's back and hangs on when the troop is on the move.

The denial of death in nonhuman primates as observed in the confined facilities of a London zoo has been described by Zuckerman (1932). He concluded that some nonhuman primates react to a dead companion as if it were alive but passive. He suggested that this reaction may be a primitive denial of death and related to the separation anxiety seen in the early stages of human bereavement.

There are, in fact, several observations of mourning among nonhuman primates and the vocalization that accompanies their grief. In the gibbon colony at the University of California (in the early 1970s), an infant died and the mother was quite distraught. During this period of mourning, the wife of a state department official in Thailand came to visit the colony because of her great interest in and knowledge of gibbons. As an associate accompanied her to the building housing the colony, she heard the vocalizations of the gibbons and volunteered that it sounded to her as if one of the gibbons was mourning. And it was! Carpenter (1940) has categorized some of these calls.

Pollock believed that chimpanzees showed the most dramatic response to death, as he cited a treatise on *Grief in Chimpanzees*, written in 1879 (Pollock 1961). After the death of a close companion, some chimpanzees attempt to arouse the dead animal, and when this fails, they manifest rage and grief. The yell of rage then gives way to crying and a plaintive moaning that seems to be intensified when the animal is left unattended. Attachment to a keeper is also common in a grieving higher primate in a zoological garden after the initial anger subsides. Observations by other workers confirm Pollock's work, for example, Garner (1900), and the Yerkes (1925; Yerkes and Yerkes 1929). Illustrated in these observations are the shock and separation anxiety stages that characterize the acute stages of grief seen in people. These observations should be instructive to veterinarians and health professionals in other disciplines in dealing with both patients and clients.

Too often our attitude toward manifestations of grief in animals is to project a kind of martyrdom because the animals display such "noble" devotion. Rather we should use these instances as opportunities to explore ways of relieving grief. We might learn much that would help us mitigate human grief as well.

The grief of Old Shep and Hachi could probably have been alleviated, at least in part, by relocating the dogs with an active individual, especially one in a similar profession as their former master and one with a similar daily schedule. If Old Shep had been relocated with another sheepherder who had appreciated him and worked with him, the dog would have been busy with his work and the grief would probably have, in part, dissipated. If Hachi had been placed with an active family that kept the dog busy during the day, or if he had been placed with a commuter, the dog's devoted activity would have been meaningful, and he would have realized some fulfillment each day with the return of the master.

The veterinarian's personal observations about the human/ companion animal bond and grief should be augmented by traditional sources of information—books, journal articles, conferences, symposia, and continuing education workshops. The need for symposia, for example, was emphasized in our opinion when we participated in one held for health professionals and social scientists. At this symposium on aging, a social scientist was describing research on the numbers of people who constitute support networks for individuals. We asked if any persons listed companion animals. The response was that such answers were disregarded. Yet on a more positive note, Schoenberg and his associates (1975) advised that grieving people should consider obtaining a pet to relieve grief. It is our hope that in future years the preprofessional and professional curricula in our schools will incorporate research on the human/companion animal bond.

Because of their professional interactions with both animals and people, veterinarians are in a unique position to relieve and prevent the grief that arises when the human/companion animal bond is threatened. At Washington State University, we are engaged in practical, community-oriented activities through the People-Pet-Partnership program (PPP) and have introduced measures that veterinarians can take to relieve or prevent grief in patients and clients (Hines 1981).

Opportunities for relieving grief of clients occur almost daily in the veterinarian's clinic or office. One of the most obvious occasions is the euthanasia of an old or ill companion animal. This situation can be intensified if the owner depends on the animal as a guide dog or hearing dog. To mitigate the resultant grief, the veterinarian should be aware of all of the possible stages and reactions to the euthanasia decision. From our experience, some of these are the following:

1. *Frustration.* The owner sees the health problems of the animal but is reluctant to part with the animal. Tension builds within the individual and within the household over the conflicting emotions.
2. *Decision.* The veterinarian presents all the alternatives to the client and a euthanasia decision is made, often precipitated by an incident emphasizing the animal's deteriorating condition. The owner is brought to realize that the animal is not enjoying life, that the greatest love the owner can show at this point is to allow the animal to be euthanized.
3. *Anger.* Children may be angry at parents and spouses may

blame each other for the euthanasia. Or they all may blame the veterinarian. The veterinarian must not return this anger in kind but show compassion and concern for an illness—grief.

4. *Sense of Loss*. For most there is a transient period characterized by crying, sleeplessness, loss of interest in everything, withdrawal and thinking of the past, weariness.

5. *Guilt*. The veterinarian often must reassure the clients that they decided rightly in not waiting, that they did not cause the illness or injury that led to euthanasia. And they should counsel the clients that they should never utter the words, "If I had only . . ." Indulging in "what could have been" is not only a useless exercise but it also intensifies an illness.

6. *Self-protection*. The clients may vacillate between the need to protect themselves from future stress by not acquiring another animal that will also die—and the need to fill the vacuum, to acquire an animal to hold, relate to, come home to.

Time and crowding in of normal activities resolve many of the dilemmas and move many clients out of the various categories described above. But the veterinarian must be alert to situations where the grief and anxiety persist and become pathological (Becker 1942; Lindemann 1944; Parkes 1974; Schulz 1975). Working with our counterparts in human medicine, we are learning how to deal with such instances.

This not only pertains at the time of a terminal illness or death of a client's animal, but also on other occasions when a client is grieving at the time of the loss of a family member, for example. Not a few veterinarians are sought out by clients to explain the meaning of the death to a child because the veterinarian is regarded as a compassionate, sympathetic, and knowledgeable friend.

A number of health professionals have indicated that a pet might aid in the relief of grief. We promote this in our PPP program. In one case, the husband in a happy marriage developed cancer that appeared terminal. He became very dejected and thought or talked only of his own problems. At one time he had owned a retriever, and it was recommended he purchase another dog. Almost immediately his interest turned from himself to the dog, and his attitude changed dramatically. Following the man's death, the dog served to ameliorate somewhat the grief of his wife, and prevent some of the dreaded loneliness of widowhood. In fact, this lady said the dog made it possible for her to continue living alone in the family home.

In somewhat the same way, parents can acquire a carefully chosen companion animal for a child who will be facing a grief period after the death of or separation from a friend or family member. Levinson (1969) has described the ways in which children not only learn to confront death through the loss of an animal, but also learn to turn to an animal for comfort when experiencing stress and grief from human losses. We believe that this strengthening of the human/companion animal bond in childhood will make it easier for individuals to turn again to animals for comfort in their old age.

The story about Sparky and his mistress does not exaggerate a situation faced daily by elderly persons. Much grief could be prevented if subsidized housing units and nursing homes would re-examine and revise no-pet ordinances. Veterinarians, as respected spokespersons knowledgeable about the real and imagined risks of zoonoses, can be leaders in changing some restrictive legislation.

Senator Eleanor Lee introduced the following bill in the 1983 Washington State Legislature:

SENATE BILL NO. 3059

State of Washington   48th Legislature   1983 Regular Session

by Senators Lee, Woody and McManus

Read first time on January 11, 1983, and referred to Committee on Social and Health Services.

AN ACT Relating to pets for the elderly and disabled; adding a new section to chapter 18.51 RCW; adding a new section to chapter 35.82 RCW; and creating a new section.

BE IT ENACTED BY THE LEGISLATURE OF THE STATE OF WASHINGTON:

NEW SECTION. Sec. 1. The legislature finds that the senior citizens of this state, particularly those living in low-income public housing or in nursing homes, often lead lonely and harsh lives. The legislature recognizes that the warmth and companionship provided by pets can significantly improve the quality of senior citizens' lives. This legislation is intended to insure that senior citizens and persons in nursing homes will not be deprived of access to pets.

NEW SECTION. Sec. 2. There is added to chapter 18.51 RCW a new section to read as follows:

(1) A nursing home licensee shall give each patient a reasonable opportunity to have regular contact with animals. The licensee may permit appropriate animals to live in the facilities and may permit appropriate animals to visit if the animals are properly supervised.

(2) The department shall adopt rules for the care, type, and maintenance of animals in nursing home facilities.

NEW SECTION. Sec. 3. There is added to chapter 35.82 RCW a new section to read as follows:

A housing authority shall permit senior citizens living in housing projects to keep not more than two pets in the senior citizens' individual housing units. Pet means a domesticated dog, cat, bird, or any number of fish contained in an aquarium.

The housing authority may adopt reasonable rules limiting the use of the common areas by pets and requiring the removal of a pet whose conduct or condition is determined to be a threat, a nuisance to other occupants, a violation of the animal's right to humane treatment, or a violation of health laws, and may adopt other rules as needed under this section. The housing authority shall not permit different terms for a tenancy based upon the presence or absence of a pet. The housing authority may relieve a tenant from liability for damages to the premises caused by the pet.

The outcome of this legislation can be the opening up of nursing homes and housing for the elderly to both visiting and resident companion animals. The results of allowing resident animals in nursing homes in our own locale have been dramatic when the elderly interact with pets (Hines 1981).

Care must be exercised, of course, in selecting the appropriate animals. Recently a research team at Washington State University wrote *Guidelines: Animals in Nursing Homes,* which details the evaluation, recommendation, and placement procedures that should be followed.

National legislation has been proposed by Representative Biaggi and Senator Proxmire that would prohibit federal assistance to rental housing projects for the elderly and handicapped if such projects do not allow tenants to have pets. If enacted, such legislation would greatly relieve grief in many persons currently in such housing, if letters we have received from across the nation are a reflection of the current unhappy situation where no-pet rules exist.

Another source of anxiety for elderly or terminally ill persons is the uncertainty of what would happen to their pets after the owner's death. This anxiety can motivate euthanasia of the pet, or can prevent the concerned person from acquiring a pet, which could bring much comfort. Our solution has been to draft an estate provision giving the animal to the PPP program to be placed in a carefully selected foster home, with costs to be paid by the estate. In at least four instances we have measurably relieved anxiety in pet owners. When the owners die we anticipate that this system will also relieve grieving in the animals.

One of the great concerns of the elderly and many who have terminal illness is the fear of loneliness, of dying alone. We feel that the presence of an animal at this time can be a great source of comfort. In one of the nursing homes in which we work, an administrator said that one of the most comforting things for some terminally ill patients is to have a loving, well-behaved cat in bed with them—something warm and furry. This ensures that they are not alone in life's most dramatic moment—the moment of death.

Pioneering in the use of animals with the terminally ill is Dame Cicely Saunders and her associates at St. Christopher's Hospice in London. They have resident animals and also allow visiting privileges to companion animals (Saunders, personal communication, 1980).

Sometimes prevention of grief can depend upon small measures. A source of great concern and distress (and grief) for the person living alone with one or more companion animals is the fear of being separated from these animals, either by having to go to a hospital or as a result of illness, accident, or natural disaster. In our PPP program, we have proposed strategies to prevent this source of concern, among them the proposal that all hospital entry forms add three questions: Do you live alone? Do you own any pets? Who is or should be taking care of them?

People who live alone or are often alone should carry a card stating the number and names of their companion animals, where they are, and who should care for them. This would relieve a great deal of anxiety should an emergency arise. In the case of a natural disaster, such as an earthquake, fire, flood, or tornado, animals are often separated from owners or owners have no provisions for keeping them. In our locality, we have established provisions for temporary housing with a supply of feed to care for animals and a message center for a source of information.

Perhaps the first and best preparation for veterinarians concerned with relieving or preventing grief in animals and people is to come to terms with their own emotions and their expression. Connected with this is the importance of facing the reality of their own eventual death and the deaths of the animals and people around them. Verbalizing and writing down one's own philosophy, as well as one's own responses when undergoing personal grief, provide a means of achieving sensitivity and clarifying values. Without a secure sense of one's own position, it is difficult to reach out to assist others.

A respected veterinary colleague said, "I have often thought of the kinship that human beings have with the rest of the animal kingdom and the veterinarian's place in expressing this kinship." He went on to say that there is a wide divergence between extreme sentimentality and a callous disregard for the rights of animals. Too many in the human race seem to regard animals as a needless intrusion in our lives. There is a middle ground in our relationship with animals, and veterinarians could and should take the lead in defining it (I. Erickson, personal communication, 1981).Part of the definition of this middle ground will include the deep attachments between animals and people that can cause grief too great for words: "Curse the sad incompetence of death." Even more critical, the definition will emphasize the human/companion animal bond that, in the words of Topsy's owner, is "one of God's sweetest gifts."

REFERENCES

Becker, H. 1942. The sorrow of bereavement. *Journal of Abnormal and Social Psychology* 27:391–410.
Bowlby, J. 1961. Processes of mourning. *International Journal of Psycho-Analysis* 42:317–40.
Bustad, L. K. 1980. *Animals, aging and the aged.* Minneapolis: University of Minnesota Press.
Carpenter, C. R. 1940. A field study in Siam of the behavior and social

relations of the gibbon. *Comparative Psychology Monograph* 16:1–212.

Garner, R. L. 1900. *Apes and monkeys: Their life and language.* Boston: Ginn.

Hines, L. M. 1981. *People-Pet Partnership program.* Alameda, Calif.: Latham Foundation.

Levinson, B. M. 1969. *Pet-oriented child psychotherapy.* Springfield, Ill.: Charles C Thomas.

Lindemann, E. 1944. Symptomatology and management of acute grief. *American Journal of Psychiatry* 101:141–48.

Lorenz, K. 1952. *King Solomon's ring* London: Methuen.

Marais, E. N. 1939. *My friends the baboons.* London: Methuen.

Parkes, C. M. 1974. Seeking and finding a lost object: Evidence from recent studies of the reaction to bereavement. In *Normal and pathological responses to bereavement,* Ed. J. Ellard et al. New York: MSS Information Corporation.

Pollock, G. H. 1961. Mourning and adaptation. *International Journal of Psycho-Analysis* 42:341–61.

Schoenberg, B. et al. 1975. Advice for the bereaved from the bereaved. In *Bereavement: Its psychosocial aspects,* ed. B. Schoenberg et al. New York: Columbia University Press.

Schulz, R. 1975. *The psychology of death, dying and bereavement.* Menlo Park, Calif.: Addison-Wesley.

Yerkes, R. M. 1925. *Almost human.* New York: Century.

Yerkes, R. M., and A. W. Yerkes. 1929. *The great apes.* New Haven: Yale University Press.

Zuckerman, S. 1932. *The social life of monkeys and apes.* London: Kegan Paul.

10

Helping
Emotionally Disturbed Children
Cope with Loss of a Pet

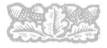

MARY LINK

It became apparent to me that the condition of the aged bay mare, Jamaica, would not improve, but it would likely be many long painful months for both the horse and the emotionally disturbed children in the riding program, before she finally died. Having her "put down" seemed the best thing to do. For 13-year old Cal, who had always ridden Jamaica and had been helping to care for her since she became ill, this news was especially hard.

HOW DO WE DEAL with the loss of an animal we have come to love? How can we help others, particularly children, deal with such losses? As the Therapeutic Riding Instructor at Green Chimneys Farm (Brewster, New York), which is part of a residential treatment center for emotionally disturbed children, I have been provided with many opportunities to search for the answers to these questions.

As I sensed Cal's need to spend time with Jamaica, and I, too, needed time to digest my decision, I put off sending her to be euthanized for a couple of weeks. Initially Cal repeatedly demanded to know why the horse had to go. Later he denied the inevitable, saying he would run away with her and cure her. He refused to let her go. He became angry, often directing his anger toward me. I allowed him to vent these feelings and he was later able to more calmly share his feelings with me of love for the horse and his pain over losing her.

During the extra time Cal spent with Jamaica, he would groom, feed, and take her for walks to graze on choice grass. He often verbalized his feelings to the horse. As the time for Jamaica to leave grew nearer, Cal began to accept that she was going and requested tokens of remembrance. I took several photographs of them together and cut and braided a swatch of her mane hair for him.

On the morning of Jamaica's departure, Cal took her for a long last walk to graze on grass, and gave her a thorough grooming. While loading her on the trailer he remarked that he had done all he could for her and was glad she was able to leave happy and well cared for. He said goodbye. After Jamaica left, Cal was unable to ride other horses for a while. He became angry occasionally and spoke of missing her. He shared his feelings with me and with other children who had cared about the horse.

Although none of the children at Green Chimneys School own the animals, they interact extensively with them on a regular basis. The therapeutic riding program provides the opportunity for all the children to care for and ride the horses. Most of the children choose a favorite horse with whom they become more involved. Consequently special friendships have also formed between children who share a favorite horse. A child may also regularly care for and develop a relationship with other farm animals such as cows, pigs, sheep, goats, or rabbits. Having urban backgrounds these children relate to the farm animals as pets more than farm-raised children might. One boy once stated while grooming his sheep, "She is like a dog to me. She knows me. Watch. She'll follow me anywhere!"

Because of the unconditional and nonjudgmental quality of the relationship with the animal, the emotionally disturbed child can take the risk involved in forming emotional attachments and can learn to trust and love. The animal friend will always listen and understand. These children believe the animal cares for them and so they feel needed, appreciated, important, and loved.

Many factors, however, can cause these almost magical relationships to be broken. Animals may die or require euthanasia because of old age or serious illness or injury. They may die suddenly from unknown causes or be killed by predators. For example sheep, geese, and rabbits have been killed by dogs. Death also enters into the midst of the joy of birth. Piglets have a high mortality rate and all extra care for a favorite runt frequently fails. Because one of the farm's roles is to produce food, an additional loss is experienced when animals are raised to be sold to market. Horses may also be shipped off to be retired or euthanized if some condition renders them no longer useful to the riding program.

Most frequently, the relationship may be broken when the children themselves leave the institution. For these institutionalized children, who have minimal control over their lives, loss from separation is comparable to loss from death. Although the children are somewhat comforted knowing that the animals will remain alive after they leave, the loss is still viewed as permanent because the children rarely return to the farm or see the animals again. Their limited writing skills keep them from maintaining contact with the farm so they are unable to check on how their animal is doing.

After witnessing the incident with Jamaica, another boy asked if he would be given similar privileges at the farm should the same thing happen to his favorite horse. I then realized that although we recognized the value and fostered the development of meaningful and therapeutic relationships between the children and the animals, we had developed no procedure for the extremely important business of helping the children deal with losses.

I then composed a series of questions related to animal loss, and several children who had recently experienced a loss or who were currently attached to an animal, were polled. A meeting of the combined farm and social work staff was called to discuss the importance of the animals to the children, to share the results of the animal loss survey, and to search for ways that the groups of staff could work together to best help the children. A proposal was discussed, that a temporary group, jointly led by a farm staff member and a social worker, be established to provide a supportive and shared experience for children with the common problems of grief, loss, and separation.

This proposed group was activated primarily as the result of a crisis situation that arose when a large horse, Jumbo, was diagnosed as having a degenerative leg disease called navicularthritis. The children's emotional attachments were jeopardized when they learned of the farm staff's decision to either retire Jumbo or euthanize him. Another reason for the immediate launching of this group of six children was the case of a boy who had taken care of a pregnant Appaloosa mare. Unfortunately the boy had to leave Green Chimneys before the foal was to be born. He was extremely anxious about leaving her and angry because he was aware that he might never be able to return to the farm to see "his" foal. The group met for a hour a week for five weeks at which time Jumbo was retired and the boy who had cared for the Appaloosa was discharged home.

Throughout the weeks that the group met, the children were allowed to spend extra time at the farm participating in special activities with their animals. A favorite and frequent activity was bathing Jumbo on hot days.

Many observations and findings from the survey, group, and experiences at the farm have added to our understanding of the loss process and have led to developing procedures for helping the children deal with their losses. In all instances of separation or death the normal stages of the loss process — denial, anger, and finally acceptance — were observed. Animal losses were comparable to human losses. Most difficult for me was dealing with the children's anger that was often misdirected at me. But as I realized that venting this often extreme, intense anger was an important and necessary part of the process for them, I did not take their anger personally and avoided becoming defensive. In cases where there was justifiable cause for the anger toward me, I attempted to accept it responsibly.

The children wanted to know about impending and sudden losses as soon as possible. Openness and honesty are extremely important and were valued by the children. Rather than unloading overwhelming amounts of incomprehensible details on the children all at once, it is better to inform them of the basics, remain available for questions, and respond when further information is requested. We also allowed the children to be involved in providing care and comfort for the animal at the time of death if they so chose. Children generally know their own limits and will usually regulate their involvement accordingly. This involvement helps them to understand and accept what is going on. An opportunity for closure with the animal is also important. The lost animal can never be replaced, but in time the child will become involved with another animal. This cannot and should not be forced. The child needs the opportunity to grieve and to then welcome the new animal. Throughout this process, a support group made up of teachers, child-care staff, and social workers was available to help the children through the transition period of losing an animal and accepting a new one.

There are several methods of helping children deal with specific types of companion animal death and separation. One method is to give the child advance notice that an animal is going to die or is going to have to leave. This advance notice helps the child work toward acceptance even before the loss occurs. We have tried to eliminate the element of surprise whenever possible. We have included the child in the process of deciding about the animal, and we have also extended the time available for closure before an animal leaves. In retiring a horse, for example, we allowed a period of time between informing the children and the actual retirement. We then arranged for extra time for the child to be involved in activities with the animal. The children have commonly chosen to feed, groom, bathe, exercise when possible, provide care when the animal is ill or injured, and throw parties for the animal. Time alone with the animal is also extremely important. By arranging this extra time we were acknowledging the importance of the relationship between the child and the animal. Also, the opportunity exists for the child to alleviate any guilt feelings, to fulfill any responsibility felt toward the animal, and to resolve any possible negative feelings directed toward the animal. The final moments shared with their animals should be successful and satisfying for the children. The chance to say goodbye to the animal is very important.

All the children who have lost animals have requested mementos of their animal, such as pictures, grooming tools, name tags, horseshoes, or tack. Most commonly requested is a swatch of the animal's hair. Interestingly, though, this only applies when the animal is still alive. There has never been a request for hair from an already dead animal.

With euthanasia and sudden or accidental death, the child should be allowed, whenever possible, to participate in or observe the arrangements being made. They may feel they must help the animal until the end, they may want to provide comfort, or they may not want to be involved at all. It is important to keep communication open and be supportive. Children at Green Chimneys have wanted to view the dead animal and participate in its burial. One boy, who was home for the weekend when his rabbit died, was furious that his rabbit had been buried without his being there. He also stated that he wanted to see the rabbit's dead body. Because children's imagination about death may be much worse than the reality, viewing the dead animal helps them to understand, acknowledge, and accept death. Participating in the animal's burial provides closure and an opportunity to fulfill a final responsibility to the animal friend. This is also an excellent time to share good memories about the animal.

Another situation we are confronted with at the farm involves the killing of production animals. Because these urban children are not as accustomed to animals being slaughtered for food as farm children might be, this issue must be addressed caringly. Prevention is the key. We have been honest and realistic about the production animals' role on the farm, and we have educated the children about where their food and clothing come from. They know not to become attached to a litter of piglets because they will all be sold. The children come to accept this. Those children who were involved with these animals were matched with other animals which were kept as breeders. Of course this preventive method is not flawless. On occasion a breeder has to go to market. We had one prolapsed ewe that could not be bred again. Because one of the children was attached to the animal, we prolonged her sale until after the child left. On another occasion a sow did not breed and the decision to slaughter her was handled as a planned separation or euthanasia. The boy chose a new piglet to keep to breed. The slaughtering and butchering of his sow were not observed.

It is important not to surprise the children with a shipping off even when they know the animals have been raised for sale. Informing them in advance gives them some feeling of control in the situation, helps to develop trust, and allows for any closure that may be needed. Generally, the children prefer to help load the animals on the truck that will take them away rather than find the animals suddenly gone.

A fourth and final method used at the farm to help children deal with animal loss was allowing a child leaving the school to train another child to care for the animal. The child feels some consolation knowing there is someone else to carry on the work that s/he had been doing with the animal.

If we believe that relationships between emotionally disturbed children and animals can be meaningful and therapeutic, then we must respect these relationships and help the children to deal with inevitable losses. When we do this, the growth potential is great. We can prevent losses where possible, prepare for losses when necessary, and provide support and caring always.

11

Development of a Social Work Service to Deal with Grief after Loss of a Pet

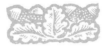

ELEANOR L. RYDER

IN OCTOBER 1978 a social work service was begun at the Small Animal Hospital in the School of Veterinary Medicine, University of Pennsylvania. As far as we could discover there was no precedent for this service. We had to establish our own structures, procedures, and methods of operation, and to engage in continuous evaluation of the usefulness of the services.

Funded by a training grant from the National Institutes of Health on Veterinary Medicine and Human Behavior, the social work was established as part of a larger operation, a Companion Animal Clinic, designed to provide services to pet owners and veterinarians on some of the human problems that emerge in a veterinary hospital, and, further, to collect data on the nature and significance of the human/companion animal bond. The clinic was staffed by graduate social services students and a postgraduate veterinary fellow under faculty supervision. The initial plan had the students working together on problems referred to them. The veterinarian was primarily responsible for problems of animal behavior and the social worker took the lead with problems of human behavior and emotion.

We began with a presentation at hospital grand rounds, in which we asked the veterinary staff to permit the clinic staff to meet with pet owners in situations where there seemed to be problems of animal behavior that could not be explained organically; where pet owners seemed to be exhibiting excessive grief, anger, or guilt; or where owners were having other kinds of problems that were interfering with veterinary practice. We thought we could learn something from these situations; we also thought we could be of help both to the veterinarian and to the pet owner.

It was apparent almost from the outset that while consultation between the social worker and the veterinarian who was dealing with behavior problems could be useful in many situations, most of the problems referred to the clinic fell primarily in the area of one or the other of these two services. They have, therefore, developed independently.

During the first year referrals to the social worker were slow in coming, and there seemed to be some feeling that the social worker might interfere with the doctor/client relationship, and/or that referral of a client to a social worker was somehow an admission on the part of the clinician that s/he was not competent to deal with client relationships. We saw few clients, and the ones we did see were for the most part people who were exhibiting extremes of neurotic or psychotic behavior. Then the Director of Oncology invited the social services students to participate regularly as a team member with the rotating veterinary students. For the first time, they had an opportunity to be in the examining room with clients, patients, and examining physicians, to observe reactions, and to offer their services to owners and veterinarians. Out of this experience the students began to identify people who might need or want to talk about their questions and concerns.

Because the hospital is a secondary care institution, we were not surprised by the depth of feeling expressed by many owners whose animals were ill. After all, people who follow up on a referral from the local veterinarian and take their pet to a university hospital have already exhibited considerable feeling for the animal and a willingness to spend time and money to restore it to health. And because most of the work in that first year was in an oncology clinic, we thought it quite natural that, although we identified a wide range of human problems and concerns, the majority of them fell in two areas: first, indecisiveness about euthanasia, with the accompanying feelings of fear, guilt and anger; second, grief, and the associated emotions, in anticipation of or following the death of an animal.

Since that first year our service has grown and has been extended to be responsive to the whole range of clinical services in the hospital. Two elements have emerged that seem to be very important: first, no matter what the area of veterinary practice, the help of the social worker is most often requested in relation to the anticipated or actual death of a pet; second, veterinarians who work with the social worker frequently recognize that their own feelings have to be taken into account as they work with disturbed clients.

I have had an opportunity to visit all of the veterinary schools in England and Scotland, to talk with clinical staff, faculty, and students about their interests and concerns related to the humans they meet in their work. The responses were similar to our experiences here: many interesting, sometimes troublesome, sometimes humorous situations arise—but consistently the most difficult to handle are those that have to do with dying and death. From this I have developed the following categorization of client problems and veterinary responses for further study:

1. Some clients treat their animals as disposable objects, and ask to have them euthanized with little expression of concern. Sometimes these are breeders who feel committed to destroying substandard animals; more often they are owners who have changed their mind about having an animal as it has grown to adulthood or who have more kittens or puppies than they can sell or give away. People who choose to dispose of an animal in this way, rather than giving it a home or turning it over to a humane society, do not seem to experience emotional difficulties about the decision. Veterinarians, on the other hand (especially veterinary students), are frequently troubled by this kind of behavior and may get quite angry about it.
2. Some clients are obviously more involved with a strong emotional attachment to an animal but are able to deal with euthanasia decisions, terminal illness, and death on their own terms. They may ask for help in thinking through alternatives in relation to euthanasia, and many are obviously glad to have an opportunity to talk briefly with either a veterinarian or a

social worker about their feeling of loss, but they do not make excessive demands. These are the clients with whom veterinarians tend to feel most comfortable, and with whom good relationships can easily be established and maintained.

3. Some clients do make excessive demands or they exhibit a variety of emotions that the veterinarian may be poorly prepared to handle. For example, a client faced with the need to choose between expensive treatment and euthanasia may be so disturbed by the situation that the reaction is one of seeming not to hear what the veterinarian is saying, and of asking repeatedly for the same information. Or the person may find it impossible to make a decision and wavers among choices. When the animal has died it is not uncommon for clients to project their anger to the veterinarian, or to become so tied up in their own guilt that they ask for repeated reassurances their decision was the right one. They may also break down in tears, threaten suicide, withdraw into silence, or become excessively verbal. All these emotions are within a normal range of grief reactions, and most can be dealt with by someone with the time, interest, and skill to work with the client. It is in this area that we have found a social worker to be most helpful.

A number of veterinarians have said to me that the thing hardest for them to respond to is tears—especially if it is a man who is crying. To that I can only respond, "How normal." Few segments of our society condone public expression of grief, especially among men, and especially for an animal. So of course we are uncomfortable when tears start streaming down the face of a recently bereaved (or about-to-be-bereaved) pet owner. Silence for listening, a friendly hand on the arm or other understanding gesture can help. One British veterinarian says, "I never know what to do, but usually I offer them a cup of tea in the back room." It's not a bad idea. I like to think it is even more helpful to be able to offer them an opportunity to talk with a social worker, or psychiatrist, or psychologist, someone who has professional skill in helping people work through painful feelings.

Peter Steinhardt (1981) has written:

We protest death in strange ways. Last summer, an anguished young lady rushed into a veterinarian's office in Redmond, Oregon. She held the patient, a decapitated ant, up to the face of the startled veterinarian and begged him to save its life. The vet, more worried about the lady than the insect, told her that he was very sorry, but without the ant's head there was nothing he could do. The lady left in tears.

Steinhardt is right, of course. It *was* a strange way to protest death. But veterinarians, involved as they are with life and death and connected as they are with the entire human component, will continue to confront strange and difficult reactions to death. As a social worker, I am glad there is so much caring, even about strange ladies with decapitated ants.

I hope what we have begun in Philadelphia marks the beginning of a long and increasingly productive relationship between professions that will provide veterinarians with new options to meet such problems.

REFERENCE

Steinhardt, P. 1981. Leave the dead. *Audubon* (January): 6.

12

Social Work in a Veterinary Hospital: Response to Owner Grief Reactions

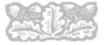

JAMIE QUACKENBUSH

THE VETERINARY HOSPITAL of the School of Veterinary Medicine (VHUP), University of Pennsylvania, has been providing social work services to pet owners for the past 3 years (Ryder and Romasco 1980). Since May 1980, in conjunction with the School of Social Work, it has been a full-time, professional service. Two of the primary goals of the social work service have been to better understand pet-owner relationships, and to provide assistance to owners distressed by their pet's medical condition. This assistance has been provided most frequently through counseling intervention by the social worker to help owners cope with their emotional reactions to euthanasia decisions or pet deaths. The manifest behaviors most typical of these owner reactions have been guilt, anger, anxiety, and depression, all of which have been observed in varying degrees of intensity and duration. It has also been assumed that the quality and depth of reaction to pet illness or loss is some measure of the degree of animal-owner attachment.

Of the 132 cases of owners referred to social work services for the year 1 July 1980 through 30 June 1981 (including 33 consultations with the VHUP clinicians) 67 percent have involved owner response to pet loss. Of the 99 referrals that required direct social work intervention, 36 percent were made for problematic owner responses to the death of a pet and 35 percent were referred for owner inability to make a euthanasia decision.

For comparative purposes it is instructive to look at the animal mortality rates for the VHUP in general as they compare with the mortality rates of the pets referred to the social work service. The present annual VHUP mortality rates for dogs and cats are 50 per 1,000 and 38 per 1,000, respectively. Those same annual rates projected for the social work service show a dog mortality rate of 459 per 1,000, and a cat mortality rate of 613 per 1,000. This is some initial confirmation that the social work service sees a significantly higher proportion of owners experiencing pet loss than would be predicted from the general VHUP population. It also supports the hypothesis that owners facing or experiencing the loss of a pet present the veterinary clinician with the greatest difficulties.

Further, we found that 80 percent of the owners referred were dog owners and the other 20 percent cat owners. Thus, compared with an annual VHUP ratio of 70 percent canine to 30 percent feline, somewhat more dog owners were referred for social work services than might be expected, but the number was not statistically significant. The data also indicate that dog size, "small dog" versus "large dog," did not play a critical role in determining owner attachment. Of the bereaved dog owners referred, 45 percent had owned small, lap-size dogs (the toy breeds), and the remaining 55 percent owned dogs too large for human laps. Again, this can be compared to the VHUP mortality figures, which show dog deaths to be 29 percent "small dog" and 71 percent "large dog." Being able to hold and cuddle a dog, then, does not appear to be something that is necessarily a major factor in developing and determining the degree of animal-owner attachment.

Pet-age and length-of-ownership data show what may be one measure of attachment. For social work referrals the mean age of dogs at death was 8.4 years. For cats, the mean age at death was 8.5 years. In the general animal population seen at the VHUP the mean age of dogs at death is 6.3 years and the mean age of cats at death is 5.4 years. A study by Dorn et al. (1967) on household pets shows a mean life span for dogs of 4.4 years and a mean life span for cats of 3.9 years. There is a tendency for the bereaved pet owners to have older animals than would be expected and perhaps this longer association is one factor that facilitates the depth and quality of the animal-owner bond. When the bond is dissolved due to pet loss, the owners of older animals give indications of needing a social work intervention more frequently than other bereaved pet owners.

Other demographic characteristics that describe this population show that 80 percent of the referred owners possessed *only* the animal presented at the VHUP, which is contrary to the multiple ownership trends suggested by Wilbur in a recent survey (Wilbur 1975). Additionally, 36 percent of these referred owners lived alone with the pet, which possibly suggests the occurrence of some of the same emotional and psychological consequences of loneliness that have been described by Lynch (1979). A final factor, that 70 percent of the social work referrals who lived alone with the pet experienced some degree of pathological grief, that is, unduly intense, delayed, prolonged, or inhibited grief (Lindemann 1944; Parkes .1965), has necessitated the primary concern of and involvement by the social work service.

With this information as a backdrop, we can elaborate specifically on the social work intervention model being used at the VHUP to help facilitate appropriate owner bereavement. The operational framework for the social work service is that of crisis intervention. Borrowing from a definition by Parad (1965), such intervention can be described as follows:

. . . entering into the life situation of an individual, family or group to alleviate the impact of crisis-inducing stress in order to help mobilize the resources of those directly affected, as well as those who are in the significant 'social' orbit. . . .

Within that definition specific methodologies, based on the Gerber (1969) model for grief therapy, are used as part of the intervention process with bereaved owners. Described previously by Quackenbush (1981), this modified pattern of intervention involves the following seven steps. It is important to understand that the sequence may vary and steps can be omitted depending on the individual circumstances of each case.

1. *Allowing and encouraging an owner to put into words and express the emotions involved in*
   (a) the pain, sorrow, and finality of the pet loss
   (b) a review of the relationship with the dead pet
   (c) the feelings of love, guilt, and anger toward the dead pet
   This initial opportunity given to the owner to express grief is particularly critical because it creates an accepting attitude and structure within which the owner may experience the loss of the pet. There exist no socially sanctioned rituals or cultural mechanisms through which grief and mourning, the interdependent components of bereavement (Averill 1968), can occur. In a sense, then, a legitimate framework for allowing the psychological, physiological, and social adaptation to the loss of a companion animal is achieved. To reinforce this statement, in postbereavement contact, more than 70 percent of the owners stated specifically that to have someone accept and understand their feelings was helpful in their efforts to resolve the emotional stress accompanying pet loss.

2. *Acquainting the owners with both the existence of and understanding of changes in their emotional and affective reactions to pet loss. Those reactions are verified as normal, natural, and necessary.*

3. *Assisting bereaved owners in finding a comforting perception of the psychic representation of the deceased pet.*
   Primarily this involves helping the owner discern and focus on the positive aspects and benefits of the relationship with their pet. They are discussed as enduring experiences always available to the owner as fond remembrances. If the owner is able to perceive the value of the relationship as being more lasting than the difficulties experienced during the animal's death, the long term response tends to be positive.

4. *Acting as a catalyst for arranging some activities for the bereaved owner, or organizing a flexible, limited schedule of activities through available, suitable family, relatives, or friends.*
   As a part of the intervention, the social worker spends whatever time necessary to educate and sensitize significant other per-

sons in the bereaved owner's social sphere to the possible emotional and psychological manifestations of pet loss. Again, this permits the owner to grieve and mourn in an accepting environment. Misunderstanding of the importance of pet-owner attachment and loss can create intrapersonal frictions between the owner and family and friends. It can also exacerbate the difficulty an owner is experiencing over a pet death.

Finally, the reaction to a pet death can temporarily impair the owner's social, psychological, and emotional functioning; support and assistance allow the owner to carry on day-to-day activities with minimal interruption. This step in the intervention process also encourages continuity in the bereavement sequence, particularly when the owner has no, or limited, outside social support.

5. *Typically, the following are avoided in the intervention:*
   (a) Explicit interpretation of key psychological defense mechanisms and emotionally laden unconscious tendencies
   (b) Excessive solicitude and overprotection of the bereaved owner

To begin suggesting psychological processes or behavior that hint at personal "abnormality" may well end in a self-fulfilling prophecy. Being psychologically vulnerable due to the pet loss means an owner is more willing and ready to believe that s/he is "crazy." A pathological interpretation of owner grief reactions is characteristically unwarranted and, with rare exceptions, inappropriate. Also, it is unwise to overstep concern for the owner as it may well discourage facing the reality of the loss, encourage excessive self-pity, and impede the occurrence of a normal grief reaction, which is a three-stage emotional and psychological process consisting of (1) shock, (2) despair and disorganization, and (3) recovery through reorganization. The owner is shown compassion, but sentimentality and overidentification are avoided. One must recognize the stress from the emotional loss but also impart the knowledge and understanding that the owner is expected to recover from the experience; a pet owner possesses and can muster the inner and outer strength to resolve the loss and return to a previous life-style. The hurt is intense and overwhelming, but it is only of limited duration.

6. *The offer of assistance in the future and a follow-up contact with the owner.*

Questions about the animal, owner feelings, and the experience of loss frequently occur after the fact. Maintaining contact for a maximum of two weeks following a pet death is the normal procedure. This includes both phone contact(s) and a written condolence. Positive owner responses to these communications indicate that the reaffirmation of genuine concern anchors and further legitimizes the owner's bereavement.

7. *Mediating referrals to a family physician or mental health professionals for antidepressants or tranquilizers and/or in-depth treatment for grief-related personal dysfunction.*

Periodically, owners have had extreme depressive reactions to pet loss: social withdrawal, insomnia, anorexia, and even suicidal thoughts (Beck 1972). Fourteen of the social work referrals at the VHUP have confirmed those types of extreme grief reactions observed by both Rynearson (1978) and Keddie (1977). The VHUP social work service is designed for short-term crisis intervention so when the possibility or need arises for an owner referral, as in the pathological grieving mentioned, owner permission is requested and required for a mental health consultation. From there, either the family physician is informed and agrees to intervene with the owner, or contact is established with an appropriate mental health program or a mental health practitioner in the vicinity of the owner's residence. By using this general approach for working with bereaved owners, we have been able to implement an owner-oriented social work service in the VHUP. This general model is also incorporated into the teaching emphasis at the VHUP which allows for the education of veterinary clinicians, veterinary students, and veterinary technicians. Through it they are better able to understand human behavior as it relates to animal attachment and accordingly approach and accommodate owners who grieve in more normal patterns.

Another result of the social work interventions has been the opportunity to examine some general animal-owner relationship patterns of bereaved owners. The data indicate at least five rather generalized, yet distinct, types of relationships. The bereaved owners had pet relationships characterized in the following ways:

1. The owner has experienced the death of at least one other significant person within the last two years: 11 percent.

The loss of a spouse, mother, father, sibling, or relative has been recent, and in all cases the pet was also owned by or cared for by the deceased person(s). Some evidence indicates these owners had not adequately resolved the human loss and that in fact they were unable to do so until the pet died. As long as the animal was alive the deceased person, at least at some psychological level, was still "alive" from the owner's perspective. The owner then seems to experience the loss of pet and human at the same time, which compounds the intensity of the bereavement.

2. The death-causing disease in the animal has been or is present in the owner and treatment procedures were identical for both: 9 percent.

These cases have involved owners and their pets having a type of cancer, blindness, or being in congestive heart failure. In addition to sharing and suffering through the same medical experience, which would seem to enhance their relationship, the owner must contend with her or his fear generated by the animal's death. That fear appears to be, simply, that of the possible outcome of their own disease process. The disease-treatment-death sequence of the animal has psychological and emotional implications for the owner whether or not the owner's medical condition justifies such implications. Ultimately the perceived outcome of the owner's illness and that impact contribute significantly to the severity of the owner's reaction to the death of the pet.

3. The death-causing disease in the animal was the same disease causing the death of a significant other person in the owner's life: 9 percent.

Here we have seen a variation on the pet-owner relationship described in the first two situations. Immediate family members and relatives of the owner have died of the disease (leukemia, heart failure, and renal failure) that caused the pet's death. Again there is the factor of the deceased person's having had a special relationship with the dead pet. At some psychological level the live pet appears to facilitate the denial of the person's death, and a final resolution of the human loss is not reached by the owner. The death of the pet, then, becomes doubly distressing because the reality of the loss of both the deceased person and the pet needs reconciliation simultaneously.

4. The pet is considered a surrogate child: 7 percent.

This particular relationship has been observed and described on numerous occasions. It is not surprising that intense, emotional reactions occur when such owners are faced with a euthanasia decision or experience the death of their pet-child. Among the human qualities they give their pets is equal life span; they never consider that animals do not live to be 65–70 human years of age. The most intense reactions have been from female owners who have never had children of their own.

5. The pet/companion relationship was strengthened as a result of the occurrence of significant periods or events in the owner's life during the ownership of the pet: 64 percent.

This final type of animal-owner relationship was the most common. The pet was very directly associated with both positive and negative incidents in the owner's personal life. That the animal was the first pet, a gift from a spouse, or purchased upon marriage are examples of positive event associations. In the situations where relationships were enhanced as a result of negative incidents, pets alerted owners to a fire, protected them from assault, and warned of an intruder. In all situations the final relationship was based on an interdependency between owner and animal as well as a common involvement in significant life events occurring during ownership.

To summarize, these preliminary social work data indicate that the development and the context of pet ownership may contribute substantially to the depth and intensity of a pet-owner relationship. There appears to be a relationship between the degree of pet-owner attachment and the association of the pet to significant life events. In particular, the ownership characteristics described above tend to accompany owner difficulty with euthanasia decisions and extreme owner reactions to pet death. The data and the conclusions, though, must be considered to be situation-and-population-specific. And as important as anything is that this group of owners represents a very small portion of all pet owners. Their reactions at best are atypical and they do not appear to represent a normative response to pet loss. To suggest they do would be misrepresentation of the data. They are a small, special population, with special needs that are beginning to be met by direct social work intervention. At a minimum, more study of this distinct population of pet owners is needed. It is clear, though, that the strength of the animal-owner bond is significant and that the breaking of the bond through death can be a stressful, debilitating experience for some owners.

REFERENCES

Averill, J. R. 1968. Grief: Its nature and significance. *Psychological Bulletin* 70(6):721–48.

Beck, A. T. 1972. The phenomenon of depression: A synthesis. In *Modern psychiatry and clinical research,* ed. D. Offer, and D. X. Freedman. New York: Basic Books.

Dorn, C. R. et al. 1967. *Zoographic and demographic analysis of dog and cat ownership in Alameda County, CA, 1965.* Berkeley, Calif.: State of California Department of Public Health.

Gerber, I. 1969. Bereavement and the acceptance of professional services. *Community Mental Health Journal* 5(6):487–95.

Keddie, K. M. G. 1977. Pathological mourning after the death of a pet. *British Journal of Psychiatry* 131:21–25.

Lindemann, E. 1944. Symptomatology and management of acute grief. *American Journal of Psychiatry* 101:141–48.

Lynch, J. J. 1979. *The broken heart: The medical consequences of loneliness.* New York: Basic Books.

Parad, H., ed. 1965. *Crisis intervention.* New York: Family Service Association of America.

Parkes, C. M. 1965. Bereavement and mental illness. *British Journal of Medical Psychology* 38:1–26.

Quackenbush, J. E. Pets, owners, problems and the veterinarian. *Compendium on Continuing Education for the Small Animal Practitioner.* In press.

Ryder, E. L., and M. Romasco. 1980. Social work service in a veterinary teaching hospital. *Compendium on Continuing Education for the Small Animal Practitioner,* 2(3)(March):215–20.

Rynearson, E. K. 1978. Humans and pets and attachment. *British Journal of Psychiatry* 133:550–55.

Wilbur, R. H. 1975. Pets, pet ownership and animal control: Social and psychological attitudes, 1975. In *Proceedings of the National Conference on Dog and Cat Control,* February 3–5, 1976, Denver, Colo.

13

Illness and Death of Pets: Role of the Human-Health-Care Team

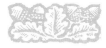

MICHAEL J. McCULLOCH

THE MANY FACTORS involved in coping with the illness or death of a pet animal create significant assessment problems for members of the human-health-care team, who must analyze and understand the human/companion animal bond in order to develop appropriate treatment interventions. The four cases discussed here illustrate this dilemma; each involves a different experience for the health professional. They demonstrate also the triangular relationship that exists among health professionals and service agencies, companion animals, and the pet-owning public.

CASE
A 7-year-old German shepherd owned by a middle-aged woman was referred by a veterinarian to a university veterinary clinic for a diagnostic workup. The dog had experienced increasing weight loss, malaise, and loss of appetite. After two days of examination, a lymphosarcoma was diagnosed. The disease was well advanced, and possibility of treatment was remote. When the veterinarian began to talk with the woman about the animal, he noted that she was very upset and tearful. Although he favored euthanasia in view of the advanced condition, he became concerned about her reaction and excused himself to call in the referring veterinarian. He explained the test results, his feelings about euthanasia, and his concern about the client's emotional state. The referring veterinarian said, "Boy, am I glad you called. I forgot to mention in my referral

that her husband died a month ago." With that information, they agreed to inform the client that her animal was very seriously ill, and that treatment recommendations had been discussed with the referring veterinarian who would carry them out when she returned home. These discussions did take place, and allowed the referring veterinarian (who had an excellent relationship with this client) an opportunity to gradually, over a 4-week period, approach the question of euthanasia. She needed this time to adjust to yet another loss.

The example illustrates a common dilemma. The client is not well known to the practitioner, and yet treatment recommendations greatly depend on knowledge of the client's emotional state and strength of attachment to the pet. In this case the veterinary practitioner was the only professional present to assess and make appropriate recommendations. It represents also a case of "double grief" and superimposed loss in which the illness and death of the animal occurs in addition to the other loss. The practitioner must be aware that in such cases the grief may be extremely intense and the emotional reaction acute. Good rapport with the client is very important, since that permits inquiry into available support systems, and may lead to phone calls to relatives or friends who can assist at this painful time. This case also illustrates that the timing of euthanasia is not always dictated by clinical evidence. It must include considerations of the pet owner's emotional well-being (Brodey 1973; Hopkins 1978). To prescribe new animals during the acute grief period is thought to be unwise, since a time of mourning is necessary (Katcher 1980; McCulloch 1978). Some pet owners elect not to have another pet; they do not want to experience another loss in the future (Wilbur 1976).

CASE

A 69-year-old woman with severe emphysema was living in an old house that had been condemned by the local health department. The woman had two dogs and many cats, and was living in a condition of utter filth. She had been contacted by the health department and told she would have to find other living arrangements. She saw her internist more frequently because of her worsening condition and now required additional oxygen at all times. Because of her concern for her animals, she consistently refused to be hospitalized and became more and more difficult to treat. Only when the internist's office nurse offered to care for the animals did she agree to go to the hospital. The condition of the animals revealed obvious improper care. After she was hospitalized it was evident she could not physically return to an independent living situation nor could she manage her own financial affairs. Psychiatric consultation was obtained. The patient's poor judgment was further confirmed. Although this woman wanted to return to living independently with her animals, all the evidence suggested this was not possible. Given the circumstances no feasible way was determined for her wish to be granted. She finally accepted a conservatorship and eventually went to a retirement center where no pets were allowed. The animals were taken to a pet adoption center where attempts were made to place them, with some success. The patient grieved very much, but gradually accepted her change of circumstance.

Numerous problems for members of the human-health-care team were addressed in this example. There were public health considerations: the patient's squalid living conditions involved numerous complaints from neighbors. This was followed by concern about the patient's mental state and ability to exercise appropriate judgment, to make proper decisions regarding her own and the animals' health. Few options were available because she clung to her insistence that she could care for her animals and herself. This case also illustrates the way in which multiple elements of the human-health-care team are drawn together to make decisions regarding very difficult situations in which pet owners are eventually separated from their pets. This is an extraordinarily difficult prospect for all concerned. Communication among members of the team is essential, and public, personal, and animal health considerations must be weighed so that reasonable decisions can be made.

CASE
    A 28-year-old woman, separated from her husband, had two dogs: a Labrador retriever and a golden retriever. They were her constant companions. She was in the process of a stormy divorce and had become increasingly dependent on the two dogs. She became very fearful when either became ill, and made frequent visits to the veterinarian. In many instances no diagnosis was made and she was simply given the reassurance she needed. The young woman entered psychiatric outpatient care at the recommendation of her family doctor because she was becoming increasingly anxious and upset about her prolonged divorce. The animals were her constant companions and at times she would bring them to the psychiatrist's office, where they sat obediently during the therapy session. A crisis occurred when the gate of her fence was inadvertently left open, and one of the dogs got loose. She became hysterical when she discovered this, and had to have a family member stay with her for several days. She was acutely distraught and grief-stricken, requiring sedation. After four days

the dog was found several miles from home and taken to an animal shelter, where it was retrieved by its grateful owner, who then realized how dependent she had become on her pets. She was then able to deal more with the reality of her impending divorce and the need to move ahead in her life.

CASE

A child, age 11, was found to have an allergy to cat dander, and a mild allergy to dog dander. He had a younger sister, age 9, who was not allergic; nor was either parent. The boy was especially attached to the dog, and his sister was much attached to the cat. The recommendation from the allergist was restrictive contact for the boy with both animals, especially the cat, and desensitization shots for the boy. The father was in favor of removing both pets and was irritated about the medical expense. The mother was supportive of keeping the pets and found herself in a mediating role. Eventually, the pets were kept, and the boy underwent desensitization shots. Several months later the cat was struck by a bicycle and its leg fractured. The family took the cat to the emergency veterinary clinic where the cost of treating the fracture was explained. The father believed this was an excellent time to get rid of the allergy problem and recommended euthanasia of the cat. The daughter was very distraught and was supported by the son. The mother attempted to mediate. The veterinarian was placed in the difficult postion of deciphering these various factors and recommending treatment. Because the family could not make a decision, they were told by the veterinarian that the animal would be sedated, and that they should go home and try to decide what course of action to take, and to call back in a few hours. The father eventually called back and said to proceed with euthanizing the cat.

When there are several members of a pet-owning family, it is very difficult at times to arrive at treatment decisions involving the pet or pet owner. In this instance treatment of the allergic child clearly had to take into account the strength of attachment, not only of the allergic child, but also of the nonallergic child. Treatment is made more difficult when family members disagree, especially because of expense. In a previous study it was emphasized that attitudes of allergists may directly influence removal of animals, even when there is not clear evidence of animal allergy (Baker 1979). In a follow-up study it was shown that 73 percent of allergic families would not get rid of pets even if it was a recommendation by the allergist. The allergists experiencing the greatest success in this area appear to be those willing to balance a clinical need for removal or decreased contact with the reality of strength of attachment between the family and the pets.

For the veterinarian the decision-making process regarding euthanasia occupies a significant portion of practice time. One study of seven veterinary practices revealed that an average of 2.1 percent or 1 in 50 contacts with the animal patients ended with a completed euthanasia. This does not take into account the amount of time the veterinarian may have to spend counseling the family, nor does it reflect the occasions in which euthanasia is considered as an alternative but other choices are made (McCulloch 1981). In many instances the family may elect palliative treatments or decide to take the pet home without treatment. Grief is a normal psychological and physiological reaction to loss or impending loss and is entirely appropriate where a strong bond has existed between pets and their owners. When a health professional encounters a bereaved pet owner, grieving should be actively encouraged as a healthy process.

For the members of the human-health-care team, understanding the nature of the human/companion animal bond is essential. As the examples have shown, many opportunities exist for health care personnel to interact with pet-owning persons. By understanding the factors influencing strength of attachment to pets, all health care professionals, physicians, veterinarians, nurses, social workers, psychologists, and others can be much more sensitive to the pet owner. The more the strength of this bond is appreciated, the more effective we can be in giving humane care to people and their animals. We should not forget our most basic obligation: to comfort when we cannot cure.

REFERENCES

Baker, E. 1979. A veterinarian looks at the animal allergy problem. *Annals of Allergy* 43:214.
Brodey, R. 1973. The pet animal with cancer. *Journal of the American Veterinary Medical Association* 162:403.
Hopkins, A. 1978. Ethical implications in issues and decisions in companion animal medicine. In *Implications of history and ethics to medi-*

cine—veterinarian and human, ed. L. McCullough and J. P. Morris. College Station, Tex.: Texas A & M University Press.

Katcher, A. 1980. Euthanasia and management of the client's grief. *Comparative Continuing Education in Small Animal Practice* 11(2):117.

McCulloch, M. 1978. The veterinarian in the human health care system: Issues and boundaries. In *Implications of history and ethics to medicine—veterinary and human,* ed. L. McCullough, and J. P. Morris. College Station, Tex.: Texas A & M University Press.

————. 1981. The pet as prothesis-defining criteria for the adjunctive use of companion animals in the treatment of medically ill, depressed outpatients. In *Interrelations between people and pets,* ed. B. Fogle. Springfield, Ill. Charles C Thomas.

Wilbur, R. H. 1976. Pet ownership and animal control: Social and psychological attitudes. Paper presented at the National Conference on Dog and Cat Control, Denver, Colo. (February) 1975.

III

Veterinary Medicine Perspectives

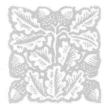

14

The Human/Animal Bond Revisited

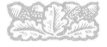

ESTHER BRAUN

THE LITERATURE is sparse in research on the human/companion animal bond, though stories abound describing these relationships. We have only to recall the tales of Jack London and the sled dogs of the North, Black Beauty and Misty of Chincoteague, Lassie and other collies in the books of Albert Payson Terhune, and the stories of mountain rescues by the famous Saint Bernards with the wine casks around their necks.

According to Konrad Lorenz (1952, 114):

> At the dawn of the later stone age, there appears as the first domestic animal, a small semi-domesticated dog, certainly descended from the golden jackal. At this time, in northwest Europe, where skeletons of these dogs have been found, . . . there is every reason to believe that the turf-dog already lived as a true house dog and that the lake dwellers had brought it with them to the shores of the Baltic Sea.
> But how did stone-age man come by his dog? Very probably without intending it . . . the stone-age hunter, for whom the large beasts of prey were still a serious menace, must have found it quite agreeable to know that their camp was watched by a broad circle of jackals, which, at the approach of a sabre-toothed tiger or a marauding cave bear, gave tongue in the wildest tones. . . . Then . . . to the function of the sentry was added that of a helper in the hunting field. . . .

The cat, birds, monkeys, cows, and many other animals throughout history have been accorded special status at different times and have interacted importantly with humans. They have been worshipped as gods, feared through superstition, sacrificed in religious ceremonies, or have simply been loved and valued as companions. Yet in a curious dichotomy, at least in Western societies, nonhuman or animal lives are counted very cheap. As Singer has written (1978, 827):

We kill animals for food, although we could feed ourselves more economically without so doing, we kill animals by the millions in our laboratories, often for trivial purposes; we kill millions more for their furs and skins, or just for the fun of killing. . . . In the East, animal life has generally been given greater consideration. Hinduism condemns the killing of animals, and strict Hindus are vegetarians. Buddhist doctrine takes a similar position. . . . Jainism . . . is even stricter than Hinduism. For the Jain, to avoid killing anything at all is the highest ideal.

In the face of such sharply conflicting tradition, it is difficult to decide how to value animal life.

From the point of view of potential benefit to humans, the human/companion animal bond, as a valuable resource, has only recently been recognized for its curative, healing, life promoting potential for troubled humans. It is also valuable to humans not necessarily in distress (Lorenz 1952, 127):

Let us admit this and not lie to ourselves, that we need the dog as a protection for our house. We do need him, but not as a watchdog. I, at least, in dreary foreign towns, have certainly stood in need of my dog's company and I have derived, from the mere fact of his existence, a great sense of inward security, such as one finds in childhood memory. . . . In the almost film-like flitting of modern life, a man needs something to tell him from time to time that he is still himself and nothing can give him this assurance in so comforting a manner as the "four feet trotting behind."

Little known or studied until now is the psychological meaning inherent in caring for and living with a pet. As the various scientific studies have shown, animals can have a unique and therapeutic value for shut-ins, people living alone, the terminally ill, the bereaved, chronically ill children and adults, people in institutions and prisons, and many others. While we all know of instances where pets have in a very real sense given an individual something to live for, a scanning of the scientific literature yields little research in studying the phenomenon more systematically. Levinson, in reporting on the use of pets in psychotherapy with children, has written, "We need imaginative and extremely rigorous research to establish principles . . . in the use of pets in psychotherapy" (Corson et al. 1977, 62). It behooves those who have used the Corson Pet Facilitated Psychotherapy, or who plan to use it, to meticulously report their studies. It may turn out that animals can be more valuable alive than dead.

Dr. Samuel Corson's innovative studies with Pet Facilitated Psychotherapy in mental hospitals, nursing homes for the elderly, and with schizophrenics and depressed patients, both children and adults, had impressively positive results. He reports (Corson et al. 1977, 61–65):

all the patients had previously failed to respond to conventional treatment and all of them showed considerable improvement . . . some of the results were startling. Patients who had refused to leave their beds, even to eat, began walking and grooming "their dog" . . . they soon made the jump to communicating with other people, and some very troubled patients have been discharged after . . . Pet Facilitated Psychotherapy. . . .

Cats and other animals (birds, even fish) have been used with success in a variety of settings. A study was conducted among elderly pensioners living alone in an urban area in Yorkshire, England. Their average age was 80 years, and many were chronically ill and withdrawn. They were offered a small Australian parrot as a pet, and those who refused to accept the parrot were given a houseplant. Among those who had taken a bird, findings (Mugford and M'Comisky 1974) indicated:

The presence of the pet . . . generally exerted a beneficial effect upon the old people's social and psychological condition. . . . Our overwhelming impression from the study is that the old people . . . had formed a surprisingly intimate (and presumably rewarding) attachment to those unsolicited pet birds . . . Not only had the bird become an object for empathy and communication in its own right, but it also had become a "social lubricant," a focal point for communication with friends, family and neighbors who came to visit.

In more conventional programs, there are the seeing-eye dogs, the "hearing" dogs, the dogs trained to fetch-and-carry for the physically handicapped, and the almost unlimited contributions of the many types of working animals on farms, especially in under-developed areas of the world. In our Pediatric Crisis Center (at Babies Hospital, Columbia–Presbyterian Medical Center, New York City), many cases of acute grief and depression reactions in children are seen following the loss of a pet.

It is often through the loss of a pet that a child first begins to learn about the meaning of death. In group meetings held for children on our wards, participants were often able to express their concerns about being ill and their fear of dying by making a peripheral reference to a pet who had been very sick or had died. Pet ownership offers children, in addition to fun, companionship, and uncritical acceptance, opportunities for learning and maturation.

In the face of recent evidence of the great potential for help to humans of companion animals of all kinds, the question naturally occurs: Why hasn't there been more utilization of this valuable resource? The study, so imaginatively carried out by Corson in 1977, had to be halted for lack of funds while there were seemingly unlimited funds for animal experiments, many of which were repetitious, poorly designed, and had little regard for the animals' suffering.

Another line of inquiry, which seems to have relevance in considering ethical issues in the relationships between humans and animals, is that of studying the intelligence and ability to communicate of various species of animals. Extensive research with chimpanzees has proved they are capable of communicating with humans by means of learned techniques, including a primitive kind of sign language. Even the frog, considered low on the evolutionary tree, is apparently able to experience anxiety. An anecdote reported by an Italian sociologist, who was watching frogs being killed for cooking, relates that just before being killed the frogs would urinate in what seemed to be anticipatory fear.

We have reached a point where we are facing a very real dilemma. On the one hand, we see animals interacting with humans as therapeutic agents and, in a multitude of ways, enhancing their lives. On the other hand, if we look at the animal research picture, we see this same creature sacrificed. Historically the wide scale experimentation on animals began in the seventeenth century "when scientific inquiries were beginning to be made in many fields," though the practice of conducting experiments on living animals goes back at least to Galen (A.D. 130–200). Descartes

(1596–1650) said that animals are "mere machines, more complex than clocks but no more capable of feeling pain." Yet Singer (1978, 79) has written:

If this convenient view of the nature of non-human animals is rejected . . . a serious ethical problem about experimenting on animals does arise, because the infliction of suffering and death on an animal seems, in itself, to be an evil.

Animal experimentation raises the issue of whether the end justifies the means and, in addition, forces us to consider what place nonhuman animals have in our ethical deliberations.

Singer estimates that in excess of sixty million animals are used in this country alone, and of these only a minority of the experiments can be classified as "medical" (Singer 1978, 80):

Many of the most painful experiments are carried out by psychologists and are intended to test theories about learning, punishment, maternal deprivation, and so on. Millions of animals are used to test foodstuffs, pesticides, industrial products, weapons, and even nonessential items like cosmetics, shampoos, and food coloring agents. . . . Many of these experiments involve severe and lasting pain for the animals. . . . In experiments on stress, monkeys have been locked into iron chairs for more than a year and made to perform tasks in order to avoid electric shock. To study the effects of heat stroke, medical researchers have slowly heated fully conscious dogs to death. . . .

While legislation governing experiments on animals varies from country to country, no law in any country prohibits outright painful experiments or requires that the experiment be of sufficient importance to outweigh the pain inflicted. The first law regulating experiments was the British Cruelty to Animals Act of 1876, which requires the use of anesthetics except where the object of the experiment would be compromised. This law is still on the books. In the United States, the Animal Welfare Act of 1970 was equally ineffectual in preventing pain and in requiring that the experiment objective be worth the cost.

Michael Ross (1978, 376, 378) has described a plan in effect in Sweden since 1976 that

provides not only for both protection and more efficient use of animals, but for improvement in experimental design and maximum availability of advisors. . . . It has been noted that simply being aware that the research has to be scrutinized before it can commence has led to improvement in research design and more research being carried out in the lower categories (painless) in preference to higher ones. . . .

In this scheme, an Ethics Committee was set up, composed of scientists, lab assistants, technicians, and lay people. Any experiment involving use of animals was submitted to this committee. It was difficult to obtain approval for those experiments that would have caused the animals the most pain. In the first year of operation, there was a sharp drop in experiments that were so classified.

Proposed in the United States has been a Research Modernization Act that would require:

— 50 percent of each agency's animal research fund be directed to the development of alternative methods of research and testing that do not involve the use of live animals
— no federal funds be used to duplicate experiments on live animals that have already been done
— programs be established to train scientists in alternative methods of research and testing that do not involve the use of live animals
— information on existing alternatives be disseminated throughout the scientific community and to the public.

It is clear that concern is increasing for the establishment of some kind of Bill of Rights for animals.

Singer (1978) views the abuse of nonhumans as a kind of "speciesism" in which we deny rights to species other than human, "a prejudice in favor of 'our own kind' that is analogous to, and no more justifiable than, racism." He questions, "Is there any ethical justification for the sharp distinction we now make between our treatment of members of our own species and members of other species?" And he asserts (p. 82) that most people concerned about the plight of animals "are united in seeking to narrow the ethical gulf that now separates humans from other animals in our conventional morality. . . ."

We enter into treacherous psychological areas when we try to find a rationale for "man's inhumanity to man" as well as humans' inhumanity to nonhuman species. We know that in the case of the

Nazis, it was first necessary to declare certain groups of individuals to be inferior, thereby relieving society of any obligation to treat their members as human beings. Historically there have been various reasons given for cruelty to animals—ranging from the religious one that animals have no soul and therefore no rights, to the Cartesian assertion that animals are merely machines. Depersonalization is an important component in the mistreatment of animals. Sperlinger (1981) has written:

Most animals who are experimented upon never achieve this mark of individuality [being given a name]—they merely have numbers and become statistics in the research data. . . . Part of learning to be "a scientist" consists of learning not to feel concerned about the effects of experimental procedures on the animals involved. . . . Part of this learning involves avoiding the language of individual feelings and relationships. The work on Animal Behavior is always expressed in scientific hygienic-sounding terminology, which enables the indoctrination of the normal, nonsadistic young psychology student to proceed without his anxiety being aroused. Thus techniques of "extinction" are used for what is in fact torturing by thirst or near-starvation. . . .

Freudian theory may possibly throw some light on the issue of human potential for cruelty not only to animals but also to fellow beings. He postulates (in *Beyond the Pleasure Principle*) a life force (Eros) and a death instinct (Thanatos) in opposition to each other. The death instinct is the organism's innate tendency to return to its simpler state, that is, its inert state or death. In its effort to defend the Ego, the life force can deflect outward the destructiveness of the death instinct. For individuals who are unable to integrate the two opposing forces, these destructive forces may seek objects upon which to vent energy. Although this may be a rather farfetched interpretation of Freud's theories, it offers a possible explanation for some of the most baffling aspects of human behavior and their pathological nature.

In 1980 thousands of signatures were collected and presented to UNESCO articulating a universal declaration of the rights of animals. Such a declaration, if enacted, would serve to raise the consciousness of people throughout the world to our ecological relationships and interrelationships with other living creatures. There is clearly a call for a change in our attitude toward nonhumans, and a message that we cease to regard as natural and inevitable our exploitation of other species. Rather, it is hoped, the moral principles established to protect human rights in a free society will be extended to protect the rights of nonhuman animals in that same society.

REFERENCES

Corson, S. A. et al. 1977. Pet dogs as nonverbal communication links in hospital psychiatry. *Comprehensive Psychiatry* 18(1) (January–February):62.
Lorenz, K. 1952. *King Solomon's ring.* New York: Thomas Y. Crowell.
Mugford, R. A., and J. G. M'Comisky. 1974. Some recent work on the psychotherapeutic value of cage birds with old people. Paper presented at the symposium, Pet Animals and Society, organized by the British Small Animal Veterinary Association, London (January).
Ross, M. 1978. The ethics of animal experimentation: Control in practice. *Australian Psychologist* 13(3) (November):378.
Singer, P. 1978. Value of life. In *Encyclopedia of Bioethics,* vol. 4, ed. W. T. Reich. New York: The Free Press.
Sperlinger D., ed. 1981. *Animals in research.* New York: John Wiley.

15

Clinical Aspects of Grief Associated with Loss of a Pet: A Veterinarian's View

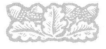

MARC A. ROSENBERG

AS A CLINICAL PRACTITIONER I see the same types of problems with pets and owners as does every practicing veterinarian dealing with companion animals. Just as every clinician is often disturbed by the torrent of emotional display sometimes associated with the deaths of companion animals, so am I. I believe if it were possible to organize the owner's grief responses in a fashion that could be easily categorized, it would certainly make my job as the supportive clinician less frustrating and the pet owner's grief state less burdensome. With the assistance of Dr. Kübler-Ross's (1969) debatable yet basically concrete observations of human adaptation to grief and the observations of fellow veterinarians, I have attempted to correlate the responses of the grieving pet owner with the emotional stages dying human patients experience: denial, anger, guilt, and acceptance.

Approximately 27 percent of the dog owners in the United States derive psychological benefits from their relationship with their companion pets (Wilbur 1976). In many cases, the pet owner's comfort and a certain amount of self satisfaction relate directly to the well-being of his companion pets. A very conservative estimate would put millions of people into this category. These psychologically linked pet owners will also experience substantial grief at the loss of these animals.

The veterinarian has been aware for decades of the magnitude of the grief associated with the loss of pets. In the past, however, the only accepted obligation that the veterinary practitioner felt was the need to cater to the comfort and well-being of his pet patient. For many years, an unwritten segregation of the veterinary and medical healing arts (in a clinical setting) was sensed by the veterinary practitioner. Physicians were generally unreceptive to unsolicited veterinary input about their human patients. Now, time and progress are starting to meld the healing arts. With a heightened awareness of the effect of the loss of companion pets on their owners (Friedmann et al. 1978), the veterinarian's last obligation to his pet patient involves dealing with the grief of the owner. This is not to imply that the veterinarian should undertake any protracted therapy involving a grief-stricken pet owner; he is neither inclined to perform this task nor qualified for it. However, a recognition of the stages of grief behavior experienced by pet owners (Katcher and Rosenberg 1978), and the classic comments almost universally uttered at these times, will allow the veterinary clinician to organize the grief observations he has repeatedly made over the years. This organization of clinical responses permits the veterinarian to further assist a pet owner at a very difficult time—a time when these people are looking for constructive support and receiving very little from those around them.

Denial, at some level, is the first stage of adaptation to the terminal state of a companion pet's health. This denial is often more pronounced in acute conditions. Denial on the part of the pet owner is demonstrated quite clearly when a clinician is confronted with a cat with advanced feline leukemia. Clinically the cat demonstrates vague signs. He is not eating well, is less active than normal, and is "just not himself." The animal is examined for what the owner feels may be a "cold" or rundown condition and the hematocrit of 9 or 10 and other obvious symptoms dictate a terminal stage of feline leukemia. When these owners are told of this condition and its options, both of which offer a poor prognosis, their agitation becomes obvious. Such remarks as, "that's impossible" and, "you must be mistaken" are also commonplace. Denial among pet owners or the hesitation to accept the reality of a terminal diagnosis may take more subtle forms.

Veterinarians are most commonly presented with the denial stage by the recounting of irrelevant information after the pronouncement of the condition. A pet owner after hearing of her pet's metastatic lung lesions may recount the dog's diet in detail and emphasize how well the dog is eating and moving his bowels. The universal phrase experienced by practitioners when dealing with owners of terminal patients is, "Doctor, would you please trim his nails?" Once again this is an owner's protective denial coming to surface.

The veterinarian must take pains not to challenge this denial because it is counterproductive. A clinician may feel s/he is not getting through to a client when these irrelevant remarks are made. When this happens, the owner is often challenged by the clinician's attempt to communicate the gravity of the situation to the client. "Mrs. Jones, you don't understand; Fluffy is dying; he doesn't need his nails trimmed." This only frustrates the clinician and sharpens the defenses of the pet owner. The client's denial will take its own course, and it may be necessary to use life-sustaining procedures for the pet patient until the owner is ready to deal with the realities of the situation.

C A S E

Gray poodle, 17-years-old. This dog was incontinent, very arthritic, had bilateral cataract development and multiple ulcerative skin lesions. The dog was presented due to the presence of a progressive cardiac cough. The owner was concerned about the cough and the fact that the dog was not eating. The pet's condition was terminal at this time.

I asked Mrs. B if the dog had been getting his Lasix and she told me she had stopped the medication because the dog "didn't need it." I told her that I felt Jet's condition was very serious and that she and her husband should consider the fact that we may lose him. Mrs. B told me that other than his cough he was doing quite well and if I felt the diuretic would help they would give it religiously. In addition she asked me about the possible removal of a papilloma on the left rear leg. I asked if they have ever talked about the fact that because Jet is quite elderly they may lose him in the not too distant future. Mrs. B responded by telling me that they had discussed this possibility but that we had to deal with his immediate problems right away. At this point, I admitted Jet to the hospital to make an attempt at stabilizing the dog's condition while the owners contemplated their pet's critical state and dealt with their denial.

As denial passes, pet owners will often begin to feel angry about their pet's terminal state. This is difficult for the practitioner because anger can also be veiled and and dispersed in many directions. Just as it is important not to confront pet owners with their denial (within reasonable limits), it is equally important not to interpret the anger stage of grief acceptance personally. Once again, many owners display this adaptive anger in subtle fashions. They may use the word kill interchangeably with euthanasia or the phrase "put to sleep." "Doc, when will you have to kill the dog?" "Do you remember when you had to kill my last dog when he got to be this age?" Most clients appreciate the meaning and starkness of the word kill in relation to a household pet, and the choice of this word is significant.

Veterinarians are familiar with obvious anger displays associated with a pet's terminal illness. Some of the more common responses are, "Why didn't you discover this sooner?" "You just don't care; it's not your dog." Although it's difficult, it is best to retain a passive, supportive stance in the face of these accusations. If they are truly valid and not just adaptive defense responses to a pet's impending death, clients will pursue their statements at a later date. This, however, rarely happens.

Feelings of guilt are not as difficult to deal with because they are not directed at the practitioner. This reaction, nevertheless, is one of anger; it is simply directed inward. "I should have come to you sooner." "We never should have let her stay in the boarding kennel last week." The pet owner will use a "retrospectascope" to ferret out any shortcomings in the care of the pet.

Rather than dwell on guilt feelings it is best to direct the owner away from this self persecution. When the clinician feels it is appropriate, anger of a hostile nature should be handled in a similar fashion. It may help to suggest that feelings of anger or guilt are not helping the pet and since the pet is the primary concern all efforts should be made to make the animal more comfortable. When the veterinarian recognizes the stages of denial and anger for what they are, s/he can remain both objective and compassionate without dealing with the frustrations these emotional responses often create.

CASE

Dr. C brought his 6-year-old Great Dane to our clinic not able to stand after having been in a kennel for two days. Complete evaluaton revealed a prolapsed lumbar disc, resulting in total paralysis of the hind legs and loss of bladder and bowel control. When this condition occurs in the giant breed dogs and is unresponsive to treatment, euthanasia is often the only humane course to follow.

Dr. C told me he shouldn't have left the dog in the kennel and he would never forgive himself for doing it. He continued to say that if the kennel had cared for the dog properly and called his veterinarian when Brutus became ill, they wouldn't have killed his dog. I mentioned the fact that they called me as soon as his dog had become "wobbly" and that a disc prolapse is often of acute onset. Dr. C told me that they would pay for their inattentiveness. The next day I received a call from an irate kennel owner asking me why I had told Dr. C that they had killed his dog. I explained that I rendered a medical opinion, and it did not include any accusation of negligence. Dr. C lost his pet and his anger; later he did not pursue his early threats.

There is nothing unique about the way a pet owner displays grief over a dying animal. This grief may even be heightened by the owner's projections of the pet's anxieties. The most remarkable facet of pet-owner grief stems from the lack of support that he gets from family and friends. The veterinarian can help this client by what I like to call "flexing expertise."

Flexing one's expertise amounts to confident reassurance based on the uncommon insight that the clinician has gained from working in these situations and the respect s/he is given by the pet owner. In interviewing pet owners who had lost dogs to whom they were very attached, it was found they were basically close-mouthed about their feelings and their pet's terminal state (Katcher and Rosenberg 1978). There is no culturally accepted method for mourning the death of a pet and because of this the grieving pet owner generally retreats into private thoughts.

In many cases, whether in person or by phone, pet owners will discuss the terminal problem with the veterinarian in an effort to get reassurance and some relief from their grief. It is not uncommon to be told, "I can't live without the dog." Owners will often dwell on the fact they don't want to lose the dog, almost as if the dog's problem is a minor consideration and their loneliness paramount. A good percentage of pet owners often speak of their concern for how their children will react to the pet's death. The veterinary clinician certainly cannot resolve an owner's grief, but s/he can now render support by flexing expertise. It helps to emphasize that the anxiety for the most part is the owner's and not the pet's. This should be a consolation in that the pet doesn't have the human fears often associated with a terminal condition. If euthanasia is an option, the clinician should support the concept that the pet owner is doing something for her or his pet and not to the animal.

TAPED INTERVIEW *(Rosenberg and Katcher 1978)*:
The B family pet died after 14 years. They told of the pain of not being able to discuss their sadness with friends for fear of being thought of as silly. Mrs. B said, we loved Pipa as a member of the family and it hurts so much to have lost her. The tears were evident as they spoke. Mr. B mentioned that he would make some excuse to get outside so he could see a similar looking dog being walked by a neighbor. This evoked a living memory of the loss of his Pipa. The B family described these classic grief feelings more than 6 months after the death of their pet.

Resolution is the stage pet owners ultimately reach when they accept the terminal state of their pet without displaying the defenses we have already discussed. This stage does not require support as much as it does recognition. The pet owner who has accepted the fact that s/he is going to lose a pet and who has moved through the earlier stages of grief usually dwells on two subjects. It is at this point that s/he will begin to solicit information about burial. S/he will show an interest in what the options for disposal of the animal are and the cost factor. The subject of another pet in the household is also mentioned. This is not discussed as a vehicle for relieving the gulf created by the condition of the dying pet, but a desire to have a new pet in the home. This should not be mistaken for the desire to replace the dying pet with one just like it. It is not unusual for owners, while severely grief-stricken, to demand help in finding a pet exactly like the one they have lost or are about to lose. Generally, during the first three stages of denial, anger, and guilt, most owners will be adamant about never again having a pet. The time necessary for a pet owner to resolve the terminal status of death of pet varies greatly. Those pet owners who have no real psychological link to their animals often won't experience the defensive stages discussed. On the other hand interviews with owners of deceased dogs have indicated that it can take 2 or 3 years for some pet owners who have become very dependent on their dogs to resolve their feelings (Rosenberg and Katcher 1978).

CASE
The G family lost a 14-year-old spaniel dog due to chronic senile deterioration. The dog was purchased the same year that their daughter was born. Rusty's death was emotionally very traumatic for Mrs. G. I casually suggested to her that she might want to think of another pet. However, I was told, "Never again, no more dogs for me."
Eleven months after the pet's death Mrs. G called. She was interested in another dog. They didn't want a spaniel but rather a retriever. She mentioned that Rusty was buried at a local pet cemetery and they appreciated the years of enjoyment he had brought. Mrs. G asked about the temperament of the retriever breed as well as the cost. She said, "It's important for us to have a dog around the house; we've had pets since we were kids."

A structural approach to the recognition of the stages pet owners experience when faced with a dying animal allows the veterinarian to be even more effective at a very sensitive task.

REFERENCES

Friedmann, E. et al. 1978. "Pet ownership and coronary heart disease — patient survival. *Circulation* 58:11–168.
Katcher, A. H., and M. A. Rosenberg. 1978. Euthanasia and the management of the client's grief. *Compendium on Continuing Education for the Practicing Veterinarian* 1(12):888.
Kübler-Ross, E. 1969. *On death and dying.* New York: Macmillan.
Rosenberg, M. A., and A. H. Katcher. 1978. Interview with owners of deceased companion pets. Unpublished data.

16

Role of the Animal Health Technician in Consoling Bereaved Clients

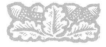

SALLY OBLAS WALSHAW

UNTIL THE MIDDLE 1960s, veterinary assistants received all their training on the job (Collins 1980). The responsibilities of these hospital attendants were limited mainly to animal husbandry and cleaning the hospital. However, technical advances introduced many diagnostic laboratory procedures into veterinary medicine, procedures which previously had been prohibitively expensive for use on animal patients. Owners began to expect sophisticated medical care for their animals. As the demands on the veterinarian's time and expertise gradually increased, they realized that skilled, trained paraprofessionals could help improve the services offered to veterinary clients. At present more than fifty training programs for animal health technicians are in progress in the United States, most of them located at 2-year colleges (Collins 1980).

An animal health technician's responsibilities can include surgical assisting, the performance of clinical laboratory procedures, animal nursing, and radiographic work. In many veterinary hospitals, technicians interact with clients while helping with outpatient examinations, answering the telephone, and assisting with the admission and discharge of animals from the hospital.

To identify the current role of the animal health technician in relation to the death of pet animals in veterinary practice, questionnaires were mailed to approximately 70 veterinarians and animal health technicians in the state of Michigan (Walshaw 1980a; 1980b). Three major areas of technician involvement with an animal's death were revealed by this survey: (1) technicians answer clients' questions about euthanasia and/or disposal of the body of a pet; (2) most technicians are required to assist with euthanasia; (3) many technicians have an active role in consoling clients who express grief over the death of a pet.

Of the veterinarians who returned the questionnaires, 97 percent reported that questions about euthanasia and/or disposal of the body of a pet animal are frequently answered by technicians over the telephone and in person. The technicians who responded to the questionnaire indicated that the usual questions asked by pet owners were: How is euthanasia of an animal performed? Is euthanasia painful? How long does it take? Can the owner be present during euthanasia? What happens to the animal's body?

All the technicians surveyed had responsibilities relating to euthanasia. In some veterinary hospitals, the technician restrained the animal during euthanasia. In other hospitals, technicians administered the drug used for euthanasia. One survey question asked in what way (if any) would the technician change her or his role with regard to euthanasia of animals in the hospital. Seventy-five percent of the respondents would not change their role. Only 8 percent would prefer never having to observe or perform euthanasia. One technician stated she would like the option to refuse participation in the euthanasia of certain animals, such as pups being euthanized for misbehavior. Another did not want to be present if euthanasia were to be performed in the presence of a hysterical owner. One technician wanted to be present if the animal to be euthanized were one she had known. Another expressed the desire to find a way to "lessen everyone's sadness" at the time of euthanasia (Walshaw 1980a).

According to both veterinarians and technicians, in at least 80 percent of the veterinary practices surveyed, animal health technicians have an active role in consoling bereaved clients. The majority of technicians — more than 70 percent — are willing to assist with consoling bereaved pet owners. However, many expressed concern over their ability to handle these situations properly.

All the respondents indicated they consider the proper handling of bereavement at the death of a pet to be an essential function of a veterinary practice. Sensitivity to this issue was exemplified by one technician who wrote that grieving clients are "allowed to cry and dab their eyes. All of us have lumps in our throats — we empathize with them" (Walshaw 1980a).

The principal technique for handling a bereaved client consisted of talking to the client. Some veterinary practices (12 percent) mailed sympathy cards to bereaved pet owners. One-fifth of the technicians reported that clients were allowed to express their grief in a quiet room in the hospital.

One of the questions asked in the survey was: Are grieving children handled differently from adults? One-quarter of the respondents stated that children were rarely present at the time of death or euthanasia. Some viewed the consolation of grieving children as exclusively the parents' duty. Others wrote that an attempt was made to explain the event to a child in terms s/he would understand.

Of the respondents, 81 percent of the veterinarians and 96 percent of the technicians believed that formal college training programs for technicians should include information on the subject of pet loss and human emotion in the curriculum. Presumably this would lead to improvements in the way veterinary hospital personnel relate to grieving pet owners. Ninety-two percent of the technicians surveyed stated that this topic was *not* included in their college training.

Technicians offered various reasons to justify including this subject in technician training programs. Some indicated feelings of helplessness in dealing with bereaved clients. ("You're really not sure what to say.") Several were concerned that inappropriate remarks could add to an owner's distress. Both veterinarians and technicians recognized that the client's respect for a particular hospital and the veterinary profession in general could be influenced by the way their grief was handled. ("If you can't communicate with these people at such a stressful time, quite often I think they get dissatisfied with the doctor, the previous care, etc.") Other respondents realized that dealing with difficult situations afforded the opportunity for personal growth. (If the technician is successful at consoling a bereaved client, "not only does the owner feel better, the technician does too.")

One-quarter of the technicians who completed the questionnaire believe that the method they are using at present for consoling bereaved clients could be improved. The major problem they identified was that the time allotted for consoling the bereaved was insufficient. One respondent cited an example of insensitivity to a client's grief as described to a class of animal technology students by a registered nurse (Franck 1980). Tearful after her own pet dog had been euthanized, she had to walk through a waiting room filled with people. She stated she would very much have appreciated a few minutes in a quiet room to regain her composure. In this nurse's opinion, a team approach with both the veterinarian and the technician involved in consoling grieving clients would be beneficial to many clients.

The veterinary profession has begun to address itself to such issues as the consoling of bereaved clients only within the past few years. It was not until the 1960s that the importance of providing comfort to dying patients and their families became widely recognized by the medical and nursing professions (Quint 1967, 11). Why has it taken so long for these issues to receive attention? Some investigators believe that part of the motivation for entering the health professions is the desire to gain control over death (Castles and Murray 1979, 11). Nursing school curricula emphasize lifesaving goals (Quint 1967, 11) and this is true also of training programs for animal health technicians.

Many people, including doctors, nurses, veterinarians, and animal health technicians, have anxieties about death. According to Castles and Murray (1979, 21), death is a "topic which many people do not know *how* to discuss, especially with an aged or dying person. Talk about death usually results in embarrassment, evasion or pretense." One explanation for the uneasiness that surrounds this topic is the fact that in contemporary American society most people die in a hospital rather than at home. Thus many young people entering the health professions have not personally known a dying individual (Castles and Murray 1979, 22; Quint 1967, 20). In

one study, only one-third of 30,000 subjects interviewed could recall from their childhood any open and comfortable discussions of
death (Castles and Murray 1979, 111–13).

Unfortunately anxiety on the part of an animal health technician regarding questions about death can result in the creation of
an emotional barricade between the technician and the client.
Nurses who withdraw emotionally from such situations do so by
using complex medical terms to avoid clear communication, by
focusing the conversation on trivial subjects, and by referring all
questions to the doctor (Castles and Murray 1979, 217–19).

Some veterinarians may question whether animal health technicians should have any responsibilities toward bereaved clients. It is
not uncommon, however, for clients to confide in technicians or
ask them to clarify specific items mentioned by the veterinarian.
This phenomenon has also been observed by nurses (Quint 1967,
145). The need for communication with a pet owner is intensified
in the impersonal and unfamiliar surroundings of a veterinary hospital. It is essential that all hospital staff members who have contact with clients be sensitive to the feelings of clients.

Although the main objective of this chapter is to consider the
role of the technician in consoling bereaved clients, it may also be
of value to discuss briefly the care that technicians can provide for
dying animals. The code of ethics of the American Veterinary Medical Association asserts that a major goal of veterinarians is the
alleviation of animal suffering. Animal health technicians can
lessen the discomfort for dying patients, as do nurses caring for
dying people, in a number of ways (Watson 1979, 15). The animal's
cage or stall can be kept clean and comfortable and, if necessary,
the animal can be helped to change position.

In one study, dying persons were asked to list the qualities that
they valued most in a nurse. These qualities included kindness, a
friendly disposition, and a genuine personal interest as evidenced
by the nurse's knowing each patient's name (Castles and Murray
1979, 222–23). These same patients reported that among the important things nurses had done were talking to them, giving back
rubs, offering water, and staying with them.

Pet animals also seem to respond to compassionate care. Pet owners (like the families of dying people) may be very sensitive to the actions of hospital personnel when a pet is dying (Blake et al. 1976, 64). It is important for the person handling the animal in the presence of the owner to be extremely gentle. It may be advisable to talk soothingly to the animal when moving it, even if it seems to be unconscious.

Some nurses advocate that family members be allowed to provide some of the care for dying patients, for example, feeding, bathing, giving back rubs (Blake et al. 1976, 66). This may help reduce a relative's guilt feelings after the person has died. The veterinary profession is increasingly able to prolong the life of animals with ultimately fatal diseases. Permitting owners to visit dying animals and to assist in providing some supportive comfort measures may be beneficial to both the owners and their animals.

Dealing with dying animals and their grieving owners is not easy. Are there any rewards for the animal health technician who is assigned such responsibilities? Many nurses believe that working with dying patients and their families gives an opportunity to gain maturity, courage, and insight into the meaning of life, pain, and death (Castles and Murray 1979, 227). Watson emphasizes that "to be human is to feel. . . . The only way to develop sensitivity to one's self and to others is to recognize and feel feelings—painful ones as well as happy ones" (Watson 1979, 16).

It is important for veterinarians to be aware of the feelings of their employees, especially if these individuals interact with bereaved clients and provide nursing care for dying pet animals. It is known that nurses grieve when human patients die, and this is no longer considered a sign of weakness (Ellis and Nowlis 1977, 364).

Depending upon the patient, the nurse, and their relationship, when a person dies a nurse may feel loss, relief, anger, frustration, sorrow, or a combination of these (Castles and Murray 1979, 230). Three main problems that may affect nurses who deal with dying patients and their families are (1) guilt feelings over the patient care or the care extended to the family, (2) feelings of inadequacy and helplessness, especially if the death were unexpected, and (3) an insensitivity to people with less serious problems (Blake et al. 1976, 69). It is reasonable to assume that animal health technicians may experience similar feelings.

Workshops and seminars on the subject of dying and bereavement have been well received by nurses who work with dying patients and their families (Blake et al. 1976, 99). Even more helpful are regular staff meetings at which feelings can be openly expressed (Blake et al. 1976, 102–5; Castles and Murray 1979, 232; Quint 1967, 161). It is generally agreed that for nurses to behave empathetically for long periods in stressful situations, they must be supported with approval, respect, and encouragement from colleagues and supervisors.

Nursing educators have recognized that mastering the technique of caring behavior is as critical a part of a nurse's education as the technological roles directed toward the treatment of physical illness. The curricula of technician training programs and veterinary schools should be examined to ensure that the subject of pet loss and human emotion is included. During training student technicians should be exposed to dying animals and their grieving owners. The objectives of such experiences and follow-up discussions are to teach the student how to (1) maintain composure with bereaved pet owners, (2) provide painless nursing care to dying animals, and (3) deal objectively with decisions related to delaying or hastening death (Quint 1967, 173). For many graduate animal health technicians, information on the subject of pet loss and human emotion will have to be obtained from veterinarian employers, continuing education programs, and a review of the available literature.

Veterinarians do not have to carry the burden of consoling bereaved clients alone. Animal health technicians, if given guidance and encouragement, are willing to assist with this task. One of the best ways of offering comfort to a bereaved client is to take the person to a quiet room and listen to what she or he has to say (Blake et al. 1976, 182; Burton 1977, 200; Quint 1967). Technicians can provide follow-up telephone calls to bereaved pet owners. Such a call may benefit the owner by allowing an opportunity to discuss the loss and to ask any remaining questions regarding the animal's illness. The effectiveness of hospital personnel in consoling a client at the time of the pet's illness and death can also be assessed during a follow-up telephone call.

Technicians should be counseled to avoid certain cliches ("he had a good life") and perhaps certain expressions, particularly the euphemism for euthanasia, "put to sleep." Painless death is a better definition of the term euthanasia. Technicians should be informed that the apparent hostility of a bereaved pet owner is usually directed against fate or the disease — not the veterinarian (Madewell 1981). Animal health technicians can help instruct lay staff members in the art of consoling bereaved clients.

Veterinarians and animal health technicians need to expand their knowledge about pet loss and human bereavement in a number of areas. They need some awareness of how death is viewed by persons of various philosophies, religions, and cultures. They should learn how to recognize the characteristics of the normal grief process, and deviations from the normal. They need to know how anticipatory grief may operate in pet owners. Guidelines are needed to help veterinary hospital personnel react appropriately to the various behaviors associated with grief in adults and children.

"Unless a person (any person, in any profession) is able to deal with death himself, he will be ill-equipped to help anyone else deal with it" (Walshaw 1980a). In a crowded, mechanized civilization the death of a pet can be a profound loss for the owner. Veterinarians and animal health technicians must accept the challenge of enhancing their skills in this important area of interpersonal relations.

REFERENCES

Blake, S. L. et al. 1976. *Dealing with death and dying.* 2d ed. Horsham, Pa.: Intermed Communications.
Burton, G. 1977. *Interpersonal relations: A guide for nurses.* 4th ed. New York: Springer.
Castles, M. R., and R. N. Murray. 1979. *Dying in an institution: Nurse/patient perspectives.* New York: Appleton-Century-Crofts.

Collins, W. E. 1980. Animal health technology: A focus on the past, present and future (Part I). *Compendium on Continuing Education for the Animal Health Technician* 1(1):6.

Ellis, J. R., and E. A. Nowlis. 1977. *Nursing—A human needs approach.* Boston: Houghton Mifflin.

Franck, C. 1980. Panel discussion on pet loss and human emotion in hospital office procedures course (VM 060), East Lansing, Mich., Michigan State University (December 4).

Madewell, B. R. 1981. Interaction with owners of cancer-stricken pets. *Journal of the American Veterinary Medical Association* 178(1):30–32.

Quint, J. C. 1967. *The nurse and the dying patient.* New York: Macmillan.

Walshaw, S. O. 1980a. Questionnaire for animal health technicians on the subject of pet loss and human emotion. Unpublished data.

_____. 1980b. Questionnaire for veterinarians on the role of animal health technicians in consoling bereaved clients. Unpublished data.

Watson, J. 1979. *Nursing, the philosophy and science of caring.* Boston: Little, Brown.

17

Owner/Pet Attachment
Despite Behavior Problems

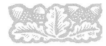

VICTORIA L. VOITH

PEOPLE show that they are attached to their pets in a variety of ways. Usually they take measures to keep pets in their proximity. Pets are often kept in the home, are taken on trips, accompany the owner throughout the day, and sleep with the owner. Some owners curtail trips or return home sooner than otherwise because a pet has been left at home. Occasionally an owner may sever a relationship with another person because that individual does not like the pet. Owners often engage in considerable effort and financial expenditure to ensure their pet a happy and prolonged life. Many owners experience grief when a pet dies and, at times, profound grief (Keddie 1977; Quackenbush 1981).

Another circumstance reflects the attachment a person has to a companion animal: many owners endure an animal's behavior problems rather than separate themselves from the animal (Voith 1981a). Owners sometimes search for ways to correct the problem, but when solutions are not readily available, many owners keep problem animals despite the inconvenience caused by the misbehavior.

A series of 100 cases seen over 4 months, December 1980–March 1981, at the University of Pennsylvania, Animal Behavior Clinic (Voith 1981b) are described below. The cases involved both dogs and cats, and the range of problems commonly seen by behaviorists (Voith 1979). The data presented were categorized according to species, breeds, and the apparent problems. Information was gathered as to whether the presenting client was living alone, was one of two adults in a household, or one of a family. A family was defined as one adult and at least one child or more than two adults. The duration of these problems ranged from several months to several years. None was of as short a duration as a few weeks. The majority of clients were asked how much of a problem the animal's behavior was to them on the following scale: *very serious, serious, not serious.* Ninety-nine percent indicated they considered the problem either very serious or serious.

The following questions were routinely asked of clients: Why had they kept the pet this long despite the problem? Had they considered euthanasia? Did they have any other pets at home? Was this their first pet?

Additionally, it was noted whether the person indicated at any time during the interview that s/he felt guilty about having caused the problem; whether the person referred to the animal as a human being in some context; and what the responses of friends and acquaintances were to learning that the client was bringing a pet to an animal behaviorist or animal psychologist for a behavior problem.

In the series of 100 cases, 61 involved a single dog, 1 involved 2 dogs in the household, 31 involved a single cat, 6 involved 2 cats in the household, and 1 case involved 3 cats and 1 dog. Sixty-two percent of these cases can be classified as dog cases; 38 percent as cat cases (the case involving the 3 cats and 1 dog was, in reality, being caused by the cats and therefore is included as a cat case). This ratio is compatible with the percentage of dogs and cats seen for medical and surgical reasons at the Veterinary Hospital, University of Pennsylvania.

Of the 61 single dog cases, 46 involved purebreds and 15 involved mixed breeds. The case involving 2 dogs involved 1 purebred and 1 mixed breed. The majority of purebred cases were represented by only one each of a specific breed. Twenty-five individual purebreds were only represented once. None of the other breeds was represented in sufficient number to indicate an overwhelming breed incidence of a specific problem.

The cat cases were made up of 27 individually presented domestic short hairs (alley cats), 4 individually presented purebreds (2 Persian and 2 Siamese), 6 pairs of cats (9 domestic short hairs and 3 Siamese), and 1 trio of cats (domestic short hairs involved in the dog and cat case). The ratio of male to female cats presented for behavior problems is approximately 1:1 and does not differ from the sex ratio of cats presented for medical and surgical reasons. The majority of dog problems involved aggressive behavior, primarily toward people. Fifty-two percent of the purebreds and 27 percent of the mixed breeds were presented for aggression. Most aggression was directed toward family members as opposed to aggression directed toward strangers. The majority of dogs were males.

The second most common problem involved separation anxiety, which can be manifested as destructive behavior in the owner's absence, excessive vocalization when the owner is gone, and elimination problems during the owner's absence. Elimination behavior problems are not always a reflection of separation anxiety and must be differentiated from elimination problems caused by disease, urine marking, submissive urination, and lack of housebreaking.

The third most common canine behavior problems were fear manifestations unaccompanied by any aggression. These fearful behaviors were primarily in response to loud noises, such as thunderstorms, but sometimes were fear of people or novel environments.

Overactivity or hyperactive behavior was the fourth most common presenting complaint. Neurological disorders, such as stereotypic flank-sucking and probable psychomotor epilepsy, ranked among the least common causes of behavior problems.

The behavior problems are listed according to complaint by owner rather than according to motivation of the animal (that is, dominance, fear, pain-induced aggression, separation anxiety), in order to better depict the problem the person had been living with.

The most common cat behavior problem was failure to use a litter box for elimination. The second most common behavioral complaint was aggression toward other cats; the third, hyperactivity; and the fourth, aggression toward people or excessive chewing behavior.

The majority of people who brought a pet in also had other

animals. Fifty-two percent of the dog owners and 68 percent of the cat owners had other pets. A smaller percentage of cases were from single households than 2 adult or family households. Only 4 of the dog owners had never had a dog before, and 2 of the cat owners had not had a cat before.

If keeping a pet that exhibits a behavior problem considered serious or very serious can be used as a measure of attachment to a companion animal, it can be seen that this attachment is not a reflection of isolation from other people. Most of the owners were living with other people. These cases show that attachment can occur between animals and people with a variety of life-styles, and independently of the ownership of other pets.

When the clients were asked why they had not gotten rid of the pet because of the behavior problem, the owners usually gave one response, sometimes two or three. The responses were categorized as follows:

1. A statement of affection, such as "I love (like) her/him," or that another person (the children, my wife) was attached to the animal.
2. Humanitarian reasons, such as "no one else would take this animal." Therefore the owners feel that they have to keep the animal or it will be put to death. "I feel that people have a responsibility to a pet," "I already saved her/his life once before" (the animal had been rescued by the person in another situation). In some cases persons expressed feeling sorry for the animal.
3. Another response category was that getting rid of the animal was not a consideration. Some owners did not directly answer the question or they had simply not considered it.
4. Other owners referred to the animal as a person and responded to the question with the statement that the pet was a member of the family.
5. Not infrequently, the owner would answer with the statement that the animal had positive attributes that outweighed the behavior problem's negative qualities. Owners would say it is a good, sweet, or lovable pet most of the time or that it is really not a bad animal.
6. Some owners answered that they thought the behavioral prob-

lem was curable; therefore they kept the animal because they thought the problem could eventually be resolved. They could not be encouraged to deviate from that specific type of answer when attempts were made to get at the more underlying cause of why they had kept the pet during the period of inconvenience.

7. Some owners answered that an animal had a monetary value.
8. Twice people answered that they could not live without the animal.
9. Occasionally, owners believed that the animal could not live without them specifically. This answer was differentiated from the answer that the animal would have to be put to sleep if this person didn't keep it because no one else would take it.
10. Although three dog owners indicated that the protective value of the dog was a reason for having kept it, this was never a first response.

Overwhelmingly, the first response (55 percent of both dog and cat owners) was a term of affection. The second most common first response (16 percent of both dog and cat owners) was a humanitarian reason. In these cases the second response was usually that of affection. The third largest category of first responses was simply the statement that getting rid of the animal was not under consideration. There were no statistical differences between any of the 10 first responses of dog and cat owners. Except for one category, there were no correlations between type of response and whether the person was from a single, 2-adult, or family household or whether the person had other pets. However, the 2 persons (1 cat and 1 dog owner) who answered that they could not live without the animal were people living alone without other pets in the household. This does not mean that all persons living alone with no other pets answered that they could not live without their pet. However, those that did give this answer were persons living alone.

There were no significant differences between the cat and dog owners as to why they kept behavior-problem pets, whether they had considered euthanasia as a solution to the problem, or whether they felt guilty about having caused the problem. There was, however, a large percentage difference in whether the owners referred to the animal as a person at some time during the session. More dog owners than cat owners (45 percent, 34 percent) referred to the pet as a person at some time during the interview. Perhaps this is because dogs have a wider range of and/or more easily recognized facial and postural expressions that result, consciously or unconsciously, in more identification with dogs than with cats.

The attachment of these owners to their pets is indicated not only by keeping pets that have problem behaviors, but also by the fact that most owners face social ridicule when they seek help from a professional behaviorist. They endure this ridicule in the hope that the outcome of the visit will make the pet a better, more enjoyable companion or, in some cases, save the animal from euthanasia.

Occasionally a person mentioned the reaction of people who learned the owner was going to take her or his pet to an animal behaviorist or psychologist because of behavior problems. The comments were generally that the pet owner was crazy, it would be a waste of money, or people merely laughed. Twenty-five persons presenting dogs were specifically asked if they had told anyone that they were bringing their pet to see an animal behaviorist or animal psychologist, and the reactions of the people they told. Fifteen (60 percent) reported a negative reaction such as "everybody laughed," "I'm a joke at the office," and "people told me *I* needed the psychiatrist." The mother of one person exclaimed, "What will the neighbors think?" Two owners said they had not told anyone. One person related how difficult it was to try and make an appointment with us without informing her coworkers. Seven owners (28 percent) reported positive reactions, and one said the information elicited no reaction.

Ten cat owners were asked the same question. Six (60 percent) reported similar negative reactions, three reported positive reactions, and one said the friend gave no reaction to the information that the owner was going to take the cat to an animal behaviorist or animal psychologist.

The above cases indicated that the attachment people have to a companion animal can be quite strong. Owners can recognize their attachment to the pet and, at the same time, acknowledge that the animal is causing them inconvenience, financial or social expenses, or emotional pain. When owners have realized that the cost or disadvantages of keeping the pet outweigh the benefits or advantages of keeping the pet, the owner will usually decide to no longer keep the pet. However, this is rarely done without regret or sorrow.

Attachment, whether defined as an emotion or strictly in terms of attachment behavior, serves to keep individuals together and as such is a mechanism for social cohesion. Attachment and/ or attachment behaviors are essential for such animals as people, canids, and equids, whose survival is benefited by sociality. People are predisposed to becoming attached to people. It is part of human adaptive strategy. Attachment and/or attachment behaviors are mechanisms to maintain social contact. In turn there are mechanisms that encourage and maintain attachment per se. Probable attachment mechanisms between people are sign stimuli, such as facial, vocal, and eye signals; length of time in proximity with each other; sharing of experiences (especially happy ones); pleasant feelings (such as joy, happiness, or love) evoked by behaviors of the other; dependency on; responsibility for; cooperative behaviors; and a tactile/contact stimulation. If attachment is a mechanism for social cohesion that in turn enhances survival, attachment should be very strong and easily evoked between parent and child.

People are primed to become attached to other people, especially their own children. Many of the attributes of children and interactions between people and children are shared by pets. The activities that serve as attachment mechanisms between people also are shared by people and their pets. Cats and dogs usually are raised by a person, and are quite dependent, even in adulthood, upon that individual. Dogs in particular have been selected for paedomorphic morphological and behavioral traits. Some breeds appear to have been neotonized. Dogs and cats engage in behaviors interpreted as being happy when the owner returns, sad when the owner departs, wanting to be touched by the owner, and looking guilty when they misbehave. Dogs and cats are capable of making the owner happy, "feeling good or feeling loved." Pets enthusiastically greet and seek out people. The animal is able to elicit guilt, especially by crying plaintively when not picked up or touched. Pets often maintain physical contact with owners for prolonged periods of time. Society allows people to touch and pet companion animals.

Since the activities that serve as attachment mechanisms between people also are shared by people and their pets, it is not surprising that people become attached to pets and relate to pets as people. This attachment persists even when the pets' behaviors pose a serious inconvenience or even threat to the owners.

REFERENCES

Keddie, K. M. G. 1977. Pathological mourning after the death of a pet. *British Journal of Psychiatry* 131:21–25.
Quackenbush, J. E. 1981. Pets, owners, problems and the veterinarian: Applied social work in a veterinary teaching hospital. In *Compendium on Continuing Education for the Small Animal Practitioner.*
Voith, V. L. 1979. Clinical animal behavior. *California Veterinarian* (June):21–25.
_____. 1981a. Attachment between people and their pets: Behavior problems of pets that arise from the relationship between pets and people. In *Interrelations between people and pets,* ed. D. Fogle. Springfield, Ill.: Charles C Thomas.
_____. 1981b. Profile of 100 animal behavior cases. *Modern Veterinary Practice* 62(6):483–84.

18

Owner/Pet Pathologic Attachment: The Veterinarian's Nightmare

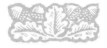

E. K. RYNEARSON

THE FUNDAMENTAL IMPORTANCE of the relationship between human and pet is reflected by its ubiquity. In every culture this bonding serves as a complementary interchange of need and satisfaction.

It would appear that this bond is based upon our commonality as animals and our mutual drive for attachment (Bowlby 1969; 1973; 1975; 1977). This drive has a neurophysiologic basis and is expressed through the predictable behaviors of caretaking and relational proximity. As ethologists have noted, attachment drive and behavior are shared by all social animal species (McGuire and Fairbanks 1977). Systematic experimentation with primates and other mammals has verified the invariable expression of attachment beginning with mother and infant. Through distinct interactional systems, which follow their own epigenesis, attachment later generalizes to include father, siblings, extended family, peers, and eventually intense male/female relationships.

I have suggested that the human/pet relationship, while biologically derived and universal, may also serve a particularized psychopathologic purpose (Rynearson 1978; 1980). The relationship becomes pathologic when the attachment interchange between human and pet assumes such significance for the human that it has greater priority than attachment interchange with other humans. In such an individual the drive for relational proximity and caretaking is displaced to the pet with such intensity that its expression is distorted into an anxious preoccupation with the pet's proximity and care.

While the sickness and/or death of a pet is always stressful to the "human members" of its family, this threat is commonly disruptive rather than calamitous. As with any process of separation and loss, the family deals with the accompanying anxiety and mourning which, while painful, are not pervasive or preoccupying. The doctor of veterinary medicine is sensitive to this dimension of psychological disruption, which can be eased through reassurance that the realistic needs for care are being satisfied and by allowing the family proximity to the pet while it recovers or dies.

This same stress of sickness and/or death of a pet creates a pathologic display of thought, feeling, and behavior in family members who are pathologically attached to the pet. The veterinarian recognizes the developing scenario in which this sort of family anxiously hovers in the clinic lobby demanding that they be near the pet. However, proximity is not reassuring, for once close there are heightened demands for not only care but cure. Under these pathologic conditions, attachment is so intense and so psychologically crucial that its threatened interruption is met with the magical expectation that the pet must somehow survive.

I know of no statistical study that describes the frequency, pattern, and outcome of this pathologic attachment and pathologic reaction to separation or loss between human and pet. That basic sort of data has eluded controlled study between humans, so it would not seem realistic to expect such study between humans and nonhumans. Clinical reports of this pathologic attachment are based on observations of dramatic clinical expression. While such observations are anecdotal and uncontrolled, they still represent significant responses.

I have a particular interest in this relationship between human and pet, and as a psychiatrist, I routinely inquire about its occurrence. I have found it to be a very productive clinical focus filled with details of much psychodynamic significance. However, I have suspected that veterinarians find themselves directly involved in what I am considering from the "distance" of my office; I have suspected that veterinarians must find themselves participant observers in this pathologic interchange which is manifest with the separation and threatened loss enforced by the illness of the pet. Whenever I have approached a group of veterinarians with my clinical interest in this relationship, they acknowledge not only its clinical occurrence but its clinical challenge:

You bet that happens and I have to play amateur psychiatrist. Those people are never satisfied no matter what happens.

One man threatened to kill me if I didn't save his dog.

This lady wouldn't leave; I wouldn't let her sleep in the clinic so she slept in her car in the parking lot so she could stay close to her cat.

Always, case after case is cited as another example of pathologic demand for proximity and care.

To present the development of pathologic human/pet attachments more clearly, consider this family with whom I worked.

The father of the patient was killed in an airplane crash two months before her birth. The mother was a fragile, immature person whose grief and detachment were so profound that she was hospitalized by her obstetrician during the last month of pregnancy. She never sought psychiatric help.

As the only child, the patient was the object of her mother's adherent attachment. The mother would cry when the patient would go outside to play, protesting that she could not tolerate being alone. Often the mother would become angry at these times of imminent separation, screaming that she was "going to die because you're leaving me." They remained in this grief-stricken symbiosis until the mother became romantically involved with a wealthy attorney. The patient was 6 at the time and remembers feeling a mixture of relief, "someone else was there to help me with Mom," alloyed with resentment and jealousy.

Shortly they married, and her stepfather became an important family figure. He was a distant person obsessed with his work, work that required travel away from home. It was his decision that the family needed a watchdog. In years previous the mother had anticipated the presence of a pet as a burdensome responsibility and had refused the patient's insistent request for a dog. Now she grimly agreed.

The patient and her stepfather selected the dog "together." While the patient wanted a small house dog, "I knew he wanted a German shepherd so I told him I had always wanted one, too." Her private wish was relinquished in an effort to please him.

The dog became her most trusted companion. He slept in her room, often in her bed, where she would hold him and share her most secret fantasies and wishes.

When the patient was 8, the school authorities recommended psychiatric evaluation to better understand the patient's marked isolation from her teachers and schoolmates. Her parents refused. They reinforced her withdrawal at home in actively accepting her isolation with her dog. The patient learned that during those frightening times when her dog became sick or strayed away, she must turn to her stepfather for support, for her mother would remain unconcerned.

The dog, though gentle and warm at home, was fiercely protective and territorial of any outside intrusion. The patient assumed the role of protective custodian, walking the dog each day on a short chain. The neighbors were frightened, but their verbal and legal complaints were gruffly ignored by the stepfather. The dog was behaving the way the stepfather wanted.

This arrangement persisted—the detached, schizoid mother; the distant, frequently absent stepfather; the patient regressively attached to the dog—until the patient was 17, when the dog bit a neighbor's child resulting in facial disfigurement and a lawsuit. The stepfather became paranoid in his defense of the dog, claiming it was "the child's fault," and a year-long legal battle ensued. By court order, the dog was finally taken from the home and sacrificed, creating a nightmarish struggle; while the patient tearfully clung to the whining pet, her stepfather screamed threats and abuses at the police officers, and the mother covered her ears and retreated to her bedroom.

Thereafter, the patient sought therapy and in subsequent treatment, which included sessions with the patient's mother and stepfather, the salient issue revolved around the patient's separation and independence. The dead dog remained an abreactive focus for the patient. Initially, it was the figure through whom and for whom she could openly express her conflicting feelings. Later, she and her mother and stepfather could focus some of these feelings on one another but only in a limited way that remained restricted by their shared distrust.

Veterinarians should be alert to the repertoire of abnormal attachment behaviors that are a common part of their practices. Their role not only involves attention to the animal, but necessarily involves the human members of the pet's family who need support at such a time.

One could be more effective in responding to the sometimes difficult demands and threats if one remembers that the basic insecurity in these individuals is one of fear and despair; beneath the façade of demands for care and proximity is a desperately frightened and despairing person. The veterinarian's professional competence is not an issue though the persistent demands often threaten that. The veterinarian can be more effective in supporting such a person if s/he remains unthreatened and empathetically focused on the owner's fear and loneliness.

It would not be realistic or appropriate for veterinarians to assume primary "care" for this frightened despairing person; that is not their job and that is not what these people want. They need to be somehow supported and reassured that the veterinarian is providing "all that can be done" for their pet. While their demands are sometimes unrealistic and insatiable, there are some practical clinical principles that might be helpful.

1. *Sufficient Time.* Support and reassurance require time and interchange. Under pathologic circumstances, announcement of the diagnosis, the prognosis, and treatment plan in a busy waiting room or corridor will be met with anxious demands. These demands can be better understood and met given 10 or 15 minutes of uninterrupted time in a quiet office. In this atmosphere there can be an interchange rather than an announcement and an opportunity to focus on some significant historical issues:

2. *Pertinent History.* How long have you had this pet? How did you find it? Has it been ill before? Who took care of it? These sorts of questions provide a clearer picture of the pet's assimilation as a family member and previous experience with the stress of sickness and separation.

3. *Social Support.* Other family members can be supportive at this threatening time, and they should be encouraged to provide proximity and caring for one another.

4. *Additional Consultation.* An additional opinion regarding diagnosis and treatment from another veterinarian can reinforce the validity of professional care. Consultation with a psychiatrist would be met with firm resistance, but referral to the family physician for medication to help manage insomnia and anxiety is usually indicated and welcomed.

REFERENCES

Bowlby, J. 1969. *Attachment and loss,* vol. I: *Attachment.* London: Hogarth.
_____. 1973. *Attachment and loss,* vol. II: *Separation anxiety and anger.* London: Hogarth.
_____. 1975. Attachment theory, separation anxiety and mourning. In *American handbook of psychiatry,* vol. 6, ed. S. Arieti. New York: Basic Books.
_____. 1977. The making and breaking of affectional bonds. *British Journal of Psychiatry* 130:201–10.
McGuire, M. T., and L. A. Fairbanks. 1977. *Ethological psychiatry: Psychopathology in the context of evolutionary biology.* New York: Grune and Stratton.
Rynearson, E. K. 1978. Humans and pets and attachment. *British Journal of Psychiatry* 133:550–55.
_____. 1980. Pets as family members: An illustrative case history. *International Journal of Family Psychiatry* 1(2):263–68.

19

Death of Pets Owned by the Elderly: Implications for Veterinary Practice

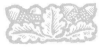

GEORGE   PAULUS,   JOHN   C.   THRUSH,
CYRUS   S.   STEWART,   PATRICK   HAFNER

THROUGHOUT THE CIVILIZED WORLD most people have been born into and died in stable communities in which the subordination of the individual to the welfare of the group was taken for granted. In contemporary American society, institutions such as the extended family and the stable local neighborhood have virtually disappeared, causing individuals to try to satisfy their affiliative needs in different ways. Twentieth-century technological change, physical and social mobility, and individualistic ethos have combined to rupture the traditional bonds that in the past tied individuals to a family and a community. These attachments provided us with a comfortable sense of social stability and self definition. For many aged in our society, these changes have meant that fulfillment of human desires for *community* (a wish to live cooperatively with one's fellows), for *engagement* (a wish to interact with one's fellow beings), and for *dependence* (a wish to share responsibility for the control of the direction of one's life) have become severely limited.

In this context, it is not unusual to find individuals seeking companionship from a pet and most pet owners become intimately aware of the psychological bond that can develop. For many elderly in our society, especially those living alone, a pet may well be the only form of companionship they have. Many researchers have provided evidence that the attachment humans develop for pets, specifically dogs, is related to the fact that most dogs have an ability to offer love and tactile reassurance without criticism (Arkov ᴠ1977; Bustad 1979; Corson et al. 1977; Levinson 1969; 1972). This, in addition to the fact that dogs maintain a sort of infantile state of innocent dependence—stimulating our tendency to offer support and protection—makes it easier to understand how and why they can become love objects.

The forces behind this People-Pet-Partnership are further illustrated in the following passage from Peale and Bradsky (1976, 178–79):

Pets are well-suited to be objects of the search for emotional certitude. Few things are as consistent and predictable as the behavior of a pet. Many devotees of pets attempt to minimize the distinction between love of an animal and the love of a person (with the help of pet food advertisements which personify animals, and which make it seem cruel not to pamper them). Some people, in fact, prefer the company of animals. One man characterized his dog as "the only living thing who really cares for me; who would be despondent if I died; who would love me no matter what happened to me in the world, or how mean I was to him." To elicit this kind of devotion, it is necessary only to feed a dog and occasionally pat it. Even when a person becomes tired or bored with the animal and ignores it, it will continue to center its life around its owner. When people find the give-and-take of normal human interaction too much to handle, having a pet may be the only emotional arrangement they can come to grips with. Pets naturally appear when human relationships are difficult to form as among the old and lonely.

The interactional structure between the pet and pet owner is portrayed in Figure 1. Each circle represents the totality of interactions for the pet and the pet owner. The intersection of the two circles represents potential specific interactions between pet and pet owner. The size of this area is principally controlled by the pet owner and will vary, in large measure, in accordance with the requirements and demands of the owner.

The size of this area is, however, also influenced both by the demands of the pet and what it can provide for the owner. The behavioral content of this interaction area thus contains such things as the actions of the owner in providing food, shelter, and protection for the pet. Coincidentally the pet provides the owner with companionship, protection, and sensual stimulation. Different types of pets are capable of providing different returns to their owner: for example, a thoroughbred horse can provide an economic return when bred, and a motor release when ridden; a dog can provide companionship, protection, and stimulation; a parakeet can provide sensual stimulation and companionship, but little protection. The size of the intersection is therefore a function of the qualities and needs of the pet owner and the pet.

Because one of the demands a pet makes on its owner is for medical care, an additional important actor enters this paradigm: the veterinarian. The role behaviors of this third actor also are represented by circles in Figures 2 and 3. The intersections, again, represent interactions resulting from the qualities and needs of the actors. For example, a pet owner requires a medical service (inoculations) for which the veterinarian receives an economic return from the owner and professional confirmation for having provided patient care.

The juxtaposition of the three interaction paradigms is presented in Figure 4. This triadic model provides a visual representation focusing our attention on the interaction that was the subject of this research.

The specifically pet-related interaction between the veterinarian and the pet owner is depicted by intersection 1 in this figure. In this area, the communication between the veterinarian and pet owner is directly related to the physical well-being of the pet. On the other hand, the interaction represented by intersection 2 has seldom been a subject of concern. Beyond the economic and advice exchange that transpires, the content of this interaction is professionally unspecified, even though there are intonations in the Principles of Veterinary Medical Ethics.

Our primary concern rests with the dynamics of interaction between two human beings at the time a pet becomes seriously ill and dies — with the role behaviors and expectations on the part of the veterinarian and the pet owner at such a time. The object of the interaction in this case is the pet owner's adjustment reactions to the absence or loss of the pet.

Given the context of human interaction among the elderly in contemporary society as previously noted, a pet's death may gener-

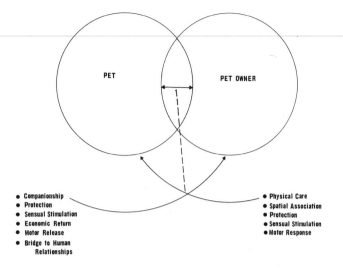

Fig. 1.   Dynamics of interaction between pet owner and pet.

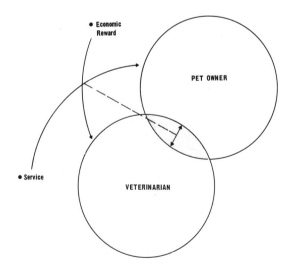

Fig. 2.   Dynamics of interaction between veterinarian and pet.

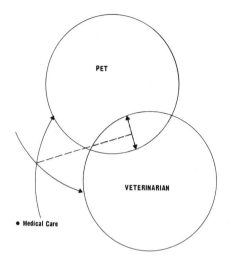

Fig. 3. Dynamics of interaction between veterinarian and pet owner.

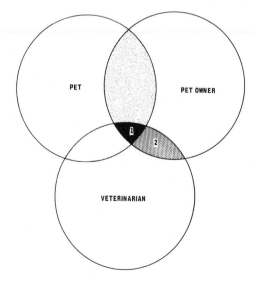

Fig. 4. Veterinarian-pet-pet owner interaction paradigm.

153

ate some serious adjustment problems that can have significant implications for the owner's physical, social, and psychological well-being. While the gerontological and thanatological literature is replete with studies exploring the dysfunctional consequences of loss for the elderly (Benedict 1973; Fell 1977; Gramlich 1968; Jeffers 1961; Parkes 1964; Prados et al. 1951; Sukosky 1977), the degree to which the loss of a pet contributes to the diminishment of self as well as the extent and potential ramifications of the pain of bereavement in such cases are empirical questions that have yet to be investigated.

Nonetheless certain studies do indicate that chronic loneliness and sudden or acute loss of significant interpersonal attachments can have a detrimental effect on healthy human functioning. In one of the most comprehensive studies to date, Lynch (1977, 181) concludes that "the lack of human companionship, the sudden loss of love and chronic human loneliness are significant contributors to serious disease (including cardiovascular disease) and premature death." Moreover the loneliness that seems to be a chronic condition of our times is strongly associated with disruptions in or absences of attachments to specific individuals and meaningful group associations (Weiss 1973).

The psychological dynamics involved in this process of chronic loneliness and acute loss of attachment bonds as preconditions for disease and death seem to focus on the manner in which interpersonal loss leads to depression. While the linkage between loss, depression, and disease is strongly suggested, the experience of loss need not be approximate in time. Studies have shown that a life-style lacking in attachment may be a present reflection of significant object loss during infancy and early childhood (Bowlby 1973). On the other side of the coin, research has shown that anxiety and other stressors produce increases in affiliative needs (Klerman 1979).

Therefore it seems reasonable to conclude that the elderly are at risk of contracting serious disease in view of their restricted relational networks and the probability of acute interpersonal loss. Even though these studies direct attention to interpersonal attachment between humans, no theoretical reason seems to exist as to why the psychological stress of object loss must be so confined. The logic seems impelling that the loss of significant attachments can be life threatening, whether the object is pet or human. If many of the elderly are as socially and emotionally isolated as recent studies have shown, then the loss of a pet can be severely traumatizing. An understanding of this relationship is a prerequisite for a better conceptualization of the role expectations placed upon veterinarians by pet owners at such a time.

When a pet is elevated to a position of affective and affiliative importance, the owner is likely to have made a significant emotional investment in the life of the pet. If the loss of this pet does generate substantial psychological stress for the pet owner, especially for the elderly, veterinarians are in a critical position to provide both support and referral assistance for the bereaved pet owner. For many elderly pet owners the veterinarian could play an important primary prevention role by assisting them in the maintenance of psychological and physical integrity after a loss occurs. The extent to which veterinarians perceive this intervention action as a legitimate dimension of their professional role is an empirical question that has not been addressed in the literature.

If, as part of their role, veterinarians do provide support to the pet owner, the additional issue of the extent to which veterinarians are prepared to provide such assistance is raised. In addition two other questions evolve from the analysis of the interaction between the veterinarian and the pet owner: To what extent do pet owners implicitly or explicitly make these support demands on the veterinarian? To what extent are these demands perceived as real by the veterinarians and considered a problem in their practices?

In an attempt to investigate the veterinarian's perception of the People-Pet-Partnership and the consequences for the elderly pet owner when such a relationship is terminated, and to identify the perceived role of the veterinarian in such situations, a survey was conducted of practicing veterinarians in geographic locations containing significant concentrations of elderly residents. A stratified, purposive sample of 375 veterinarians in Florida and Arizona was drawn from a list of currently licensed veterinarians practicing in counties containing the highest ratio of elderly residents (65 years or older). In October 1979, questionnaires were sent to the selected sample, with a follow-up to the nonrespondents in November. Two-hundred-nine veterinarians returned usable responses; 6 veterinarians responded that they no longer had an active practice and chose not to participate. An additional 10 returned unusable questionnaires (they indicated their practice was exclusively equine and therefore chose not to participate). Five veterinarians were unlocatable because of address changes and the questionnaires were not forwarded by the Post Office. The total usable responses ($n = 209$) represents 55.7 percent of the original universe. The potential sampling bias generated by this rate of return is minimized by the characteristics of the respondents. The characteristics directing the original stratification were: time in practice, small animal practice, and elderly clients.

The responding veterinarians were equitably spread throughout the time-in-practice spectrum. Forty-three percent of the veterinarians had been in practice for 5 years or less, 25.4 percent from 6 to 10 years in practice, and 31.5 percent reported having practiced for 11 or more years. A predominant number of the respondents had a small animal practice. Eighty percent reported that their practice was "almost exclusively a small animal practice." An additional 12.4 percent reported that their practice was 51 percent to 75 percent small animal, and the remaining 7.6 percent indicated that less than 50 percent of their practice was devoted to the care and treatment of small animals. A sizable proportion of the responding veterinarians' practices involved service to elderly pet owners. Twenty-four percent of the veterinarians reported that 40 percent or more of the pet owners for whom they provided service are approximately 65 years or older. Thirty-one percent indicated that from 20 percent to 40 percent of their practices dealt with pet owners approximately 65 years or older, and the remaining 44.5 percent reported that 20 percent or less of their practices involved dealing with elderly pet owners.

At a 1980 conference, we reported that 86 percent of a sample of elderly pet owners indicated their major reason for owning a pet was the companionship these animals provide (Stewart et al. 1980). This group consistently reported that they believed elderly pet owners, regardless of their marital status, have a moderate-to-strong psychological dependence on their pets. In addition, this elderly sample reported a strong belief that the death of an elderly owner's pet might result in ill health for the owner.

Based on this research, it is important to see the degree to which veterinarians, the third party in our interaction paradigm, hold similar perceptions of the elderly's psychological dependence on their pets. The data provide consistent support for the finding that both elderly pet owners and practicing veterinarians believe the elderly are dependent on their pets. Our sample of practicing veterinarians believed that the majority of elderly widows have a *moderate-to-strong* psychological dependence on their pets (95.2 percent). The veterinarians also indicated a belief that a great majority (90.9 percent) of elderly couples are dependent (defined as *moderate-to-strong*) on their pets. Almost 8 of 10 veterinarians in our sample (79.9 percent) believed that elderly widowers are dependent on their pets. While elderly widows are believed to have the greatest dependence on their pets, it remains clear that, like the elderly themselves, practicing veterinarians believe that a sizable proportion (88.7 percent) of the elderly, regardless of marital status, have this strong dependence.

Veterinarians believe the elderly perceive their pets in substantially human relationships. In fact, almost 9 of 10 (87.1 percent) veterinarians have the impression that "for elderly pet owners the status of their pet is close to that of a human family member."

Given the consistency of the veterinarian's belief that, regardless of marital status, the elderly are significantly attached to their pets, and that they elevate this relation to a human level, it is important for us to analyze the role behaviors of the veterinarians surrounding the death of an elderly person's pet. (Since our analysis revealed that marital status of the elderly was not a specifying variable for veterinarians, it will not be considered in subsequent analyses.)

In light of the perceived People-Pet-Partnership relation, the death of the animal will likely cause the grief and bereavement reactions that usually attend the loss or death of a loved one (Parkes 1964). The veterinarians in our sample seem very sensitive to this reaction on the part of the elderly. This sensitivity is revealed by the 63.6 percent who *agree* or *strongly agree* with the statement, "In general, it is more difficult to tell an elderly owner than a younger owner that his/her pet has died." The probable basis for this perception is that younger pet owners have a more elaborate relational network and, therefore, do not depend so heavily on relations with the pets as the elderly do. This seems suggested by the fact that almost three-quarters (73.7 percent) of our veterinarians agree that "the death of an elderly pet owner's pet might result in a state of ill health for that owner."

In view of the human-family status of the elderly's pets, the perceived probability of illness consequent to the death of a pet, and the perceived difficulties veterinarians have when telling an elderly pet owner that her or his pet has died, the veterinarians' response to this situation is very surprising. Although the above perceptions may be valid, they do not seem sufficient to stimulate follow-up inquiries by the veterinarian. The survey revealed that only 10.6 percent of veterinarians always or almost always "follow-up the death of an elderly pet owner's pet to see how they are adjusting to this loss."

One explanation may be that veterinarians believe that the impact of the death of a pet for an elderly owner is not an aspect of their professional identity or, alternatively, veterinarians may feel willing but professionally unprepared to assume this responsibility. The extent of psychological dependence evidenced by elderly pet owners does place a burden on the veterinarian, since 77.5 percent of our sample felt this weight of responsibility. Moreover, 83.7 percent of these practicing veterinarians *disagree* or *strongly disagree* that the personal difficulties resulting to elderly pet owners when their pets die are *not* a professional issue for practicing veterinarians. In view of their belief that this is an issue that should concern the veterinarian, the low percentage of respondents who actually follow-up the death of an elderly pet owner's pet to see how the owner is adjusting to the loss lends credence to the possibility that this discordance is based on the veterinarians' feeling of being unprepared to deal with personal adjustment to traumatic loss.

The feeling of professional unpreparedness is strongly indicated in the responses received. While not restricting themselves to any specific age category, a majority of our sample veterinarians (82.3 percent) *agree* or *strongly agree* that they "would benefit from formal exposure to some type of experience that would familiarize them with the psychological effects the death of a pet has on its owner." Almost one-half (45.5 percent) of those who desired some style of formal exposure indicate a preference for continuing education. More than one-quarter (26.8 percent) would like to see the impact of pet death on its owner be the subject of empirical research in professional journals. Only 11.5 percent indicated a preference for conferences or workshops on this subject. These data provide impelling evidence that the hesitation of veterinarians to follow-up pet death is a function of their feeling of professional unpreparedness; a feeling they express a strong willingness to do something about.

The focus of the research reported in this paper has been three-fold:

1. the perceptions that veterinarians hold regarding the psychological dependence of elderly pet owners on their pets
2. the implications of this dependence for the professional role behavior of veterinarians
3. the veterinarians' perceived need for professional death education

Based on a survey of veterinarians practicing in geographical areas with large concentrations of elderly residents (Florida and Arizona), it is evident that these veterinarians perceive elderly pet owners to be significantly dependent upon their pets. The extent of this psychological attachment is revealed by the veterinarians' belief that the pet of an elderly owner is a "family member" and that the pet's death can have significant implications for the health status of the owner.

Given the overwhelming agreement by the sampled veterinarians of the negative impact of pet death for the elderly, it was interesting to find that the veterinarians' behavior was dissonant with their perceptions. Our data reveal that the basis of their hesitancy to act was not a function of their perception of their professional role. In fact a majority of the veterinarians sampled directly indicated that the personal problems that might develop as a result of the dependent relationship (the People-Pet-Partnership) between elderly pet owners and their pet(s), particularly at the time of their pet's death should be a professional concern of practicing veterinarians. The implications of the above go beyond pet death to the general psychological reaction of separation anxiety suffered as a consequence of the loss of significant objects (Broden 1970; Peretz 1970). Specifically, the veterinarians should become sensitized to those situations where elderly pet owners experience any type of loss related to their pet (for example, stolen or runaway).

Recent literature indicates that the veterinarian can play a significant role in primary prevention of human stress and overall human therapy (Arkov 1977). Not only have investigators discussed the implications of "pet therapy" for individuals in stress situations (prisoners, for example), conditions of loss (grieving pet owners), and human loneliness, but also for mental health therapy (the mentally retarded, learning disabled, and emotionally impaired) (Bustad 1979).

Realizing that many constraints prevent the addition of death education to what is already a tight curriculum in veterinary medicine, it is apparent that an appropriate response would be to deal with this area within the framework of continuing education. The present research reveals a high level of receptivity for continuing education experiences that would enhance the veterinarian's ability to meet the demands of the situation of loss and separation. This position is supported by the fact that the sampled veterinarians were strongly in favor of this potential new dimension of their professional role.

A veterinarian attuned to the potential ramifications of loss, sensitized to the signs of reactions to grief, and knowledgeable about the significance of support structures should be capable of providing direct or indirect assistance (through referral to community and/or family support systems) to pet owners as they move through the bereavement process.

REFERENCES

Arkov, P. 1977. Pet therapy: A study of the use of companion animals in selected therapies. American Humane Association, Washington, D.C.
Benedict R. 1973. Living conditions and everyday needs of the elderly with

particular reference to social isolation. *International Journal of Aging and Human Development* 4:179–98.

Bowlby, J. 1973. *Separation: Anxiety and anger.* New York: Basic Books.

Broden, A. 1970. Reaction to loss in the aged. In *Loss and grief: Psychological management in medical practice,* ed. B. Schoenberg et al. New York: Columbia University Press.

Bustad, L. K. 1979. How animals make people human and humane. *Modern Veterinary Practice,* 60:707–10.

Corson, S. A. et al. 1977. Pet dogs as nonverbal communication links in hospital psychiatry. *Comprehensive Psychiatry* 18:61–72.

Fell, J. 1977. Grief reactions in the elderly following the death of a spouse: The rise of crisis intervention in nursing. *Journal of Gerontological Nursing* 3:17–20.

Gramlich, E. P. 1968. Recognition and management of grief in elderly patients. *Geriatrics* 23:87–92.

Jeffers, F. C. 1961. Attitudes of older persons toward death: A preliminary study. *Journal of Gerontology* 16:53–56.

Klerman, G. L. 1979. The age of melancholy? *Psychology Today* 12(11):36–42, 88.

Levinson, B. M. 1969. *Pet-oriented child psychotherapy.* Springfield, Ill.: Charles C Thomas.

———. 1972. *Pets and human development.* Springfield, Ill.: Charles C Thomas.

Lynch J. L. 1977. *The broken heart: The medical consequences of loneliness.* New York: Basic Books.

Parkes, C. M. 1964. Effects of bereavement on physical and mental health: A study of the medical records of widows. *British Medical Journal* 2:274–79.

Peale, S., with A. Bradsky. 1976. *Love and addiction.* New York: New American Library.

Peretz, D. 1970. Reaction to loss. In *Loss and grief: Psychological management in medical practice,* ed. B. Schoenberg et al. New York: Columbia University Press.

Prados, M., K. Stern, and G. Williams. 1951. Grief reactions in later life. *American Journal of Psychiatry* 108:289–94.

Stewart, C. S., et al. 1980. The elderly's adjustment to the loss of a companion animal: People-pet dependency. Paper presented at third annual conference of the Forum for Death Education and Counseling, St. Louis.

Sukosky, D. 1977. Sociological factors of friendship: Relevance of the aged. *Journal of Gerontological Nursing* 3:25–29.

Weiss, R. S. 1973. *Loneliness: The experience of emotional and social isolation.* Cambridge, Mass.: MIT Press.

20

Psychosocial Model
of Veterinary Practice

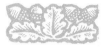

WILLIAM H. SULLIVAN, CAROLE E. FUDIN

THE MODEL of a veterinary practice, the Cat Practice, described in this chapter, attends to the physical and emotional needs of pets and their owners. It considers the importance of providing a homelike rather than hospitallike setting, and offers an approach in which the veterinarian and her or his assistants make up a health care team. The team encourages the formation of a supportive and empathic relationship with the client. With the team's example and help, the client is able to be an active participant in providing emotional and medical support for the sick and/or dying pet.

The aim of the health care team is to provide professionalism with compassion. Formality is eschewed; the health care team is known on a first name basis, and its performance is directed toward maintenance of a personal relationship.

The veterinarian, generally, is alone considered by the client as the professional member of the team, the one person to whom medical questions or behavioral problems should be addressed. At the Cat Practice, the emphasis has been placed on training members of the team to be able to respond to fundamental client queries, to be able to pass on information knowledgeably and concisely to the veterinarian. Thereby the team should be able to provide a degree of comfort and reinforcement to a client who may be in a state of distress. Client questions about bowel movements, vomiting, urination patterns, eating habits, and emotional status are routine.

In addition to the veterinarian the health care team consists of a hospital administrator, several laboratory technicians, and veterinary assistants. The latter group serves as receptionist, nurse, and medical or laboratory assistant, as required. This system allows for greater mobility in staffing. Work hours are staggered to accommodate personal schedules and professional needs, as in the case of designated surgery hours and hospital patients who require around-the-clock nursing.

Consultation with a psychotherapist for behavioral/emotional problems affecting both human and animal clients opens another dimension of the health care team, and addresses a need too often ignored in veterinary medicine. A therapist who is particularly attuned to the psychosocial aspects of human/animal stress related to disease, death, and bereavement can be an invaluable asset to the veterinarian. This collaboration can help to structure a practice, environmentally and emotionally, to better meet the needs of all served and to reduce stress as much as possible. In addition to being a referral source for clients experiencing acute or morbid grief reactions, the consultant can help the veterinarian and staff to comprehend client dynamics, thereby assisting them to expand their sensitivity to client issues during the period of pet care. This serves to reduce staff stress by providing a person with whom anxieties and fears in handling specific situations can be discussed: the hostile client, the demanding client, the fearful client.

A therapist well versed in thanatology (the psychology of terminal illness, death, and bereavement) can aid in providing death education to clients who experience difficulty in discussing or approaching the subject. For example, many clients have children and are concerned about their child's ability to cope with the loss of a pet, which may be the child's first experience with death. The therapist/consultant can tell parents how to approach the subject with children of varying developmental ages. Helpful reading materials can be suggested (including appropriate stories about animals who have died), which parents and children can read and discuss together.

Resident cats and long-term boarders play a special role in the team concept. Clients respond spontaneously to them and come to know the cats by name. They provide them with the affection they need and this interaction concurrently provides the client with an opportunity for sharing and affection as well as relieving some unrecognized tension. Stroking and talking to an animal, as has been illustrated in numerous examples of animal therapy with the ill and aged, can be as supportive as a human hug.

Resident cats play an unique role in Cat Practice–client communication. Cards are sent routinely to clients, advising them of the need for an annual examination or a special visit, such as biyearly cardiogram. These cards, cut from colored paper in the shape of a cat, and often illustrated by a member of the health care team, are addressed to the pet and inscribed as follows:

Dear Ruby: Tuesday, please have your mom make an appointment for you. It's time for your annual checkup. See ya soon! Renfield.

The cards provide the kind of personal touch that also serves to make a visit to the veterinarian a pleasant experience, rather than an arduous one. They may be sent as a follow-up to a serious pet illness ("Glad you're back on your feet again!"), or simply to follow-up a visit ("You're sure looking spiffy!").

"The Cat Practice, Good Morning, David Speaking," is the typical greeting from the phone receptionist. This approach provides the client with a personal reference to the staff (David) and offers initial expression of warmth. If the client calling has a specific problem, this information is relayed to the veterinarian, and an appropriate course of action is initiated. If the client is calling to make an initial appointment, a basic yet concise information form is completed by the receptionist, and the appointment is confirmed.

At the time of the client's first visit, a thorough medical history is taken by a member of the health care team; coffee or tea are offered as well. The procedure is similar to that which a human patient experiences on the first visit to a physician. It serves to establish the personal relationship with the client in a quasi-social environment.

During this procedure the cat remains in the carrier to avoid any distractions. This time for recording the medical history allows the client to share feelings about the cat's condition — including personal observations of habits, behavior, and any deviations from established patterns and routines—and enables the veterinarian to better understand the role that the pet plays in the client's life. Supportive listening, along with questioning and encouraging the client to express views and feelings, will form the foundation of a trusting relationship with the veterinarian and the health care team. This information also contributes to the formation of a psychosocial profile of the client, her or his homelife, the pet's behavioral patterns within that context, and the quality of the client/pet relationship.

Another section of the history asks specifically whether there is any increased stress in either the pet's environment or the client's life. Stress is an important factor in many feline diseases—asthma, feline urinary syndrome, and idiopathic eczema, for example. This discussion may elicit fears, real and imagined, that the client has not been able to articulate. It is not unusual for a female client to mention that she is pregnant, or planning to become pregnant, and may require or request specific advice about toxoplasmosis, thereby allaying some fears as to how cats and babies live together.

Specific questions are posed about any changes in the cat's behavior or attitude toward the client, and if companion cats are treating this animal differently. Often a positive, normal relationship between companion cats will deteriorate when a healthy animal perceives an occult disease, such as hypertrophic cardiomyopathy or feline infectious peritonitis, in its companion. This will lead to the shunning and persecution of the afflicted cat. Cats are excellent diagnosticians in this respect.

During the physical examination it is important that both client and patient are relaxed. Catnip, gentleness, stroking, and talking softly can help the cat. The veterinarian's stethoscope quickly loses out to a little mound of catnip on the examination table, from the pet's point of view. The client is aided by knowing there is no need to restrain the pet; stroking and soothing will suffice. Performance anxiety can result if the client feels the need to handle the animal, when the client may, indeed, be in an anxious state, and can transmit this anxiety to the animal.

Talking through the steps of the examination is done whenever possible. Saying, "Well, the liver and spleen feel normal," brings the client a step closer into the procedure, and serves as reassurance that the examination is proceeding normally.

When the medical situation requires hospitalization for the pet, communication and the medical team concept become particularly important. The more information provided to the client, the easier it is to understand the need for hospitalization. When a radiograph has been taken it is important it be shown to the client and compared to a normal example. This often makes it easier for the client to comprehend the severity of the situation and the need for hospitalization.

All veterinarians are familiar with clients whose attachment to their pets is perhaps their most meaningful, cathected relationship. Upon even a brief separation, their fears become overwhelming and they may become hostile or demanding, or appear to completely disregard or misinterpret information relayed by the health care team. Such clients will ask the same questions repeatedly, and in general may become extremely trying to even the most patient veterinarian and team. In many of these cases a verbal recognition of their underlying fear and a supportive hand may be enough to ease them through the hospital procedure. At this time, when hospitalization is imminent, a member of the health care team will join the veterinarian and client — usually the hospital nurse, who will take the client back into the wards.

Clients are encouraged to see where their cats will be during the hospital stay, as it allays fear of the unknown. We also encourage clients to leave some personal belonging, like a glove or handkerchief or the towel from the carrier, in the nook with the cat. Familiar smells help relieve the anxiety generated by unfamiliar surroundings.

The nurse now writes up the admission record. S/he may ask if the cat has eaten, and what are its favorite foods. Once all the necessary information is obtained, the nurse asks if the client would like to spend some time with the pet. People deal differently with separation anxiety. Some will want to leave the cat quickly, while others will need some time for stroking and talking. This too can be soothing and therapeutic for both cat and client.

In many chronic but manageable disease processes the burden of treatment is placed on the client. We assume our clients are responsible and believe they can be helped to cope with the pet's problem and assist in the treatment, even if that means inconvenience. For example the owner of a diabetic cat must be made aware that daily insulin injections and surveillance will be necessary. But the emphasis should be placed on the healing, that this is an opportunity to preserve and protect a valued life.

The health care team spends the necessary time instructing and teaching the client the required procedures and techniques, and follows up by telephone, especially in those first few difficult days at home. With this support and the expectation of this support, fewer people will opt for euthanasia rather than treatment.

Evaluating the client/pet relationship and understanding the home situation are necessary in order to assess the client's ability to cope with the pet's continuing health problem. This information will have been gathered during the history taking, the physical exam, and subsequent client contact. Input from members of the health care team, nurses, for example, is valuable because people will often act differently with different staff members.

Before chronically ill cats are released from the hospital, one of the nurses or the hospital director discusses the diagnosis, prognosis, testing procedures, and results with the client. Specific instructions in administering medication, whether pills or injections, are written down and discussed with the client at the time of release. The veterinarian is available for questions, but generally the nurse already has answered them thoroughly.

Clients are encouraged to call with any additional questions or problems. By this time, a familiarity has been established between the client and members of the health care team, and there is confidence that both client and pet will be recognized readily when calling with an inquiry or progress report. Follow-up phone calls or cards extend the feeling of support to the client and prevent feelings of abandonment.

We believe some people may decide upon euthanasia inappropriately, not because of the cost of pet care or a lack of concern for the animal, but because they are fearful that they alone won't be able to meet the needs of the ill cat. By extending the team support to their homes, we often give people and animals meaningful time together that otherwise they would not have had. This also allows the client to come to terms slowly with the pet's illness and, if death is imminent, provides the chance to experience anticipatory grief.

Often, animals are brought in in serious condition. In an emergency the animal needs immediate veterinary assistance, and client communication must be limited and secondary. Here the health care team is particularly effective in dealing with client needs. While the veterinarian, the nurse, or the assistant are treating the pet, the receptionist will talk sympathetically to the client, offering coffee or tea, and returning periodically to the treatment room to bring out a progress report. It is important the client not be isolated or ignored at this time. The client is under a maximum amount of stress. There may be guilt about delaying the visit, or human contribution to an animal accident. Fears about death may be very intense, and the client may need to ventilate these feelings. Tactile interaction – a hug, a pat on the shoulder – serves as vital reinforcement and bridges the isolation perceived by the client to exist between the waiting room and the treatment area.

If the animal cannot be saved, the quality of this communication assumes greater significance. It is incumbent upon the health care team member to be candid and compassionate, so that the client's trust remains intact and the client is able to relate rationally in a highly charged emotional situation. Attempting to assuage client feelings by vague statements – so as not to "upset" the client – only serves to intensify client anxiety and create a false sense of security. Truth is the best, the only tack.

If the animal is stabilized and can be admitted to the hospital, it is often valuable to ask the client to remain and help monitor fluid drip or breathing. This gives the client a sense of contribution to the pet's care. A half hour of this participation may assuage some of the guilt and relieve feelings of helplessness and dependency. Having the client support and soothe the critically ill pet for a short period under supervision will often aid the pet in unfamiliar surroundings, relieve client fears, and partially free some of the hospital staff.

The client is encouraged to call and visit the hospital as much as possible. Severely stressed cats will stop eating; the client may be asked to bring favorite foods and toys to help coax the cat into taking nourishment. Visits are soothing to the cat by bringing familiarity to strange surroundings, and the client once again feels like an integral member of the health care team. Depression and stress in both client and cat may be eased or prevented by encouraging such interaction.

Supporting an animal and its owners during the procedure of euthanasia can be as rewarding as achieving a medical or surgical coup. But, if it is to be accomplished successfully, the procedure requires comprehension by the veterinarian of the emotional range of responses possible in the client and confidence in her/his own feelings and attitudes.

Practitioners may feel at times inadequate and frustrated when faced with terminal disease processes. If these feelings result in a brusque, authoritarian attitude, the impact on the client can be devastating. The client's questions will remain unanswered, guilt will predominate, fears will remain undispelled, and emotions battered.

Likewise if a triage mentality prevails ("Well, on with the living and savable patients"), clients' needs are grossly unsatisfied and the risk is greater that the veterinarian will be blamed for the illness and concomitant medical procedures.

Obviously, in many situations requiring euthanasia, it is appropriate to proceed without delay, but in some of these cases the pet may be given an analgesic so that the client has time to assimilate the situation. This humane and compassionate approach gives the client a chance to express fears, reservations, and concern, and enables the client to share in the experience. Indeed, even if all medical procedures have been exhausted, the ultimate authorization for euthanasia must come from the client, and the client must have the opportunity to prepare for this decision.

Certain general principles will help in dealing with the stress of euthanasia:

1. It is important to have a consistent and defined hospital policy concerning animal rights. At the Cat Practice, we do not declaw, and we make clients aware of this at their first contact.

We believe the animal's rights are as important as the client's rights. Our stated position on euthanasia is that it requires:
— a confirmed diagnosis of a terminal, unalterable disease
— a patient who is suffering or no longer has a quality of life
We try to make the client aware of our euthanasia policy as soon as euthanasia becomes a possibility. By establishing such policies we can meet our clients' expectations more consistently. Predictability tends to decrease stress.

2. We must try to understand specific situations of our clients. We must listen, record, and appreciate the constraints under which they are functioning. This appraisal of the client's life situation is essential so as to know how to present options. Often the same disease process may call for a different thrust of recommendations, depending upon the general emotional, health, financial, and familial situations of the client.

3. Understanding the nature of the client/pet bond is critical in presenting options correctly. A good example of this is the older cat dying slowly of chronic renal failure. We believe that letting the cat die at home is every bit as reasonable as euthanizing the pet when activity and appetite fall off. The client's life situation and the nature of the client/pet bond would determine the recommendations. Through a careful history, and the development of a personal relationship, the health care team will have enough information about the client and pet's relationship so that we can present options without causing feelings of guilt in the client.

An example of this is a client whose cat had a dangerous tumor. Although euthanasia was an alternative, chemotherapy with uncertain outcome was another. From discussions with the client it had been learned that her mother had died of terminal cancer only a few months before, and that the client was morbidly afraid of chemotherapy because she had blamed her mother's terrible condition late in the disease on this treatment, rather than on the cancer. Obviously it was valuable to have this information when outlining the options for treatment of the pet.

4. The last general principle in reducing stress is full disclosure. If the health care team has spent some time with the client discussing test results and patient progress, the groundwork had been

laid for sensitive discussion about euthanasia. A client who is made knowledgeable about the specifics of the disease situation has usually had time to assimilate the fact that the disease may be irreversible.

Discussions about euthanasia are better conducted in person. The telephone can serve as a barrier to emotional expression, and expression of feelings is what should be encouraged. A visit to the hospitalized pet generally is advised. Sometimes just seeing the withdrawal of a pet will bring home the message that the situation is hopeless and will be painful.

Clients will signal their ability to deal directly with euthanasia. Some may need time to come to terms with it, and when possible they should be given as much time as they need. If the cat is suffering greatly, it may be necessary to impress this fact upon the client in an attempt to speed up the process of working through feelings. The death of any loved being can trigger old feelings about prior losses. Clients may need to talk about other animals they have lost, deaths of important people in their lives, or about their feelings regarding death in general. All these issues may be important to bring forth a peaceful resolution of the painful present.

A most important step after the client has decided on euthanasia is to supportively ease the client through the procedure. There are those people who want nothing to do with it. Nonetheless it is important that the entire health care team treat this event as meaningful. Although euthanasia is common in our practices, it is an uncommon and extremely powerful experience for most people. Research indicates that many people have continuing problems with the death of a pet because family, friends, and society in general do not judge it as an event worthy of much grief. We have euthanized cats of teenagers and young adults who could not remember life without the pet. These are very special bonds, and it is important to legitimize these feelings of grief. The veterinarian can tell clients shortly after euthanasia that s/he, too, shed many tears after euthanizing one of her or his own cats, and how it hurt for many weeks. Such an approach makes clients less reticent to show strong feelings.

Recognizing the effectiveness of nonverbal communication is a key element. Words are not always adequate to convey meaning, and more often than not a gentle touch or a hug is far more soothing than any word of compassion.

It is also important to discuss what the cat's death may mean to a companion cat left behind. Grief reactions in cats are quite common. In two separate cases, cats who lost a longtime companion cat progressively cut down on their activity and eating and drinking. Then slowly, after several weeks of their owners' attempts to boost their morale by extra attention and affection, it became apparent that they were getting worse. Physical exams, blood and urine tests, and X rays were all within normal limits; in one case, the cat's situation was so bad that exploratory surgery was performed. All tests were negative.

This client was perfectly willing to bring a kitten home for the cat. The improvement was instantaneous and permanent. The cat became more active, less restlessly vocal, gained weight, and returned to normal.

The owners of the other cat were much more resistant to the idea of introducing a new cat, but agreed to the offer of the "loan" of a young cat as a trial. The cat's improvement was not as rapid as in the first case, but very noticeable after several days, and the clients decided to keep the foundling.

Advising the client of possible grief reaction may accomplish two things. We may better prepare the client to deal with a possible health problem, and also suggest that the client's own feelings of grief are both legitimate and normal.

Once euthanasia has been decided upon, it is very important to schedule it for a calm time of the day. At the Cat Practice, this would be at the end of office hours, about 9 P.M. In this way, the client does not have to feel rushed or unduly pressured. It is critical for the client to have time to express any doubts, ask questions, or merely share some extra time with the pet before the euthanasia.

If clients choose to participate, it helps to reduce their stress to detail the sequence of events with precision, and to explain their role in the procedure. We give our clients an option about involvement, but encourage active participation. We believe the support and comfort they can provide the pet is critical to the pet's ease, as well as to the client.

Participating in the euthanasia enables the client to see the process as an essentially gentle procedure, thereby eliminating any fantasies about suffering and painful death. Participation reinforces the reality of death and facilitates grief casework. Furthermore, knowing that one's pet met death in a supportive environment with people who cared is a powerful and meaningful event that soothes human conscious and unconscious fears about dying alone.

Generally the client and the veterinarian are seated. Catnip is placed inside a face mask, and the cat is given nitrous oxide and oxygen for several minutes. With the client and veterinarian gently stroking the cat, the anesthetic agent is staged up very gradually until the cat is anesthetized. Usually the cat loses consciousness without any excitement at all. When the cat is completely anesthetized, the fatal injection is given.

The client is prepared prior to administering the fatal injection. The kinds of responses the animal may have are explained, and reassurances are given that the animal will not feel pain. The client is given the option of stepping outside for a few moments or staying until the end. Most clients elect to stay.

When the animal is dead, the veterinarian and client spend some time together. The client may continue to stroke the pet. Often, client and veterinarian have cried together, and this is mutually beneficial. The client is offered some time alone with the pet for a last goodbye.

All clients are sent a condolence letter about a week after their pet's death. The letter encourages them to call if they need any further assistance. Some clients are contacted by phone if they are perceived to have an especially difficult time adjusting to their loss. On occasion condolence letters have brought responses from clients who were dealing with their pet's death in unhealthy ways, ways which the health care team did not anticipate.

One such client, Miss S, a 31-year-old woman, had a cat suffering from kidney failure. She brought Linus in when he already was gravely ill. We had not known the client prior to this visit. She was a nervous, guarded woman who clearly had a deep attachment to her cat. When the cat was hospitalized, Miss S was somewhat suspicious of hospital procedures but did not protest. When encouraged to talk about her feelings, she seemed amazed and continued to close the door to communication.

Linus died in the hospital. She saw the cat after his death, did not show much emotion, paid her bill and left.

In response to a condolence card, she called. She expressed confusion about the card, and ventilated anger about how her Linus was alive but being kept for experimental purposes. She had developed a full delusional system about her cat, but willingly accepted an appointment to come in and see that Linus was not there.

A special time was set aside for her. She was taken through the hospital and shown that her cat was gone. Although she acknowledged that Linus wasn't there, she wondered if the cat had been hidden from her or sent to an experimental laboratory. When the veterinarian acknowledged her feelings — that it was hard to believe her Linus was gone — she began to express a little grief. She was asked if there was anyone in her life to whom she could talk about her relationship with Linus, and she said she had no one. Her mother viewed her attachment to the cat as peculiar and was even relieved that Linus was gone. Her deep sense of aloneness was shared by the health care staff, and it was supportively suggested that it might help if she talked to someone who would be particularly sensitive to the importance animals have in our lives. This would help her to feel less alone and give her an opportunity to talk openly about what it meant to live with and without Linus. Although hesitant, Miss S accepted a referral to the psychotherapist who serves as an extension of the health care team. While she planned to make only one visit, she found that she could talk about Linus and really begin to deal with his loss. In time, she was able to begin to explore the feelings of loneliness, isolation, and lack of love that she had felt throughout her life in her human relationships. She has a long way to go, but has made a wonderful beginning.

This last example helps to illustrate the role of the psychotherapist/thanatologist as consultant to a veterinary practice.

As has been described, the suggested model for veterinary care employs a health care team approach, in a homelike environment, and provides support both to the pet and its owner. Collaboration with a mental health professional who is particularly versed in thanatology is also recommended.

Although these concepts have been used in a practice exclusively devoted to cats and their owners, the model could be incorporated into many kinds of veterinary practices.

21

Family Psychotherapy Methodology: A Model for Veterinarians and Clinicians

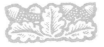

D. T. WESSELS, JR.

THE PHENOMENON of professional burnout seems to be examined increasingly in current psychotherapy literature. Briefly, *burnout* is attributed to a clinician's failing to attend adequately to her or his own needs, while trying continually to be a resource to the patient. The symptoms of burnout are depression, waning enthusiasm for work, and a prevailing sense of futility (Larson et al. 1978).

How burnout influences clinical work might be described as follows. A clinician enters a therapeutic relationship with the expectation, either consciously or unconsciously, that s/he can effect positive change in the patient. The clinician, to some degree, measures success by changes noted in and reported by the patient. The more vulnerable clinician is the one who has a *high* expectation of change in the patient. In times of high anxiety in the clinical setting, therefore, the vulnerable clinician is likely to become overly helpful, advice giving, and produce more interpretation than a less vulnerable clinician. Also, s/he fails to listen quietly to the patient. Through demeanor, the vulnerable clinician is likely to feed her or his anxiety back to the patient, thus frustrating therapy. Not only are the patient's efforts thwarted but the clinician comes to see her or his efforts as failing, which adds to anxiety, and so the pattern repeats.

While this phenomenon may say something about the clinician's overvaluing work as a source of self-esteem, it also may say something of how s/he approaches work. In the example cited the vulnerable clinician views professional effectiveness as being able to change behavior in another person. Such a myopic view of therapy negates environmental, genetic, and motivational factors affecting patient change. In essence the vulnerable therapist assumes responsibility that belongs to the patient. S/he also sets expectations (to change the patient), that are beyond her or his ability to control.

In an effort to counter burnout, the vulnerable clinician can approach the problem from two aspects. The first is evaluating what is missing in her or his life that results in the overvaluing of work. While this aspect is a realistic concern, it is too nebulous to be addressed here. The other approach to burnout is to develop a realistic definition of one's professional responsibilities. This implies defining success in terms of one's own behaviors (to render good treatment is reasonable; to cure or correct a patient's problem may not be). The clinician who consistently renders good treatment is likely to have a higher cure rate than one whose quality of treatment is inconsistent. However, this does not imply a direct cause and effect relationship. To judge one's quality of treatment as to whether a cure was effected leads the clinician to frustration and discounts the importance of numerous extraneous factors.

While my comments thus far pertain to the field of psychotherapy, I believe a similar phenomenon operates in the veterinary setting. In developing stress management training for veterinary clinicians, I interviewed numerous veterinarians. From these discussions, it became clear that veterinarians perceived more stress in trying to relate positively to anxious pet owners than in performing medical treatments for the pets. Specifically veterinarians reported more anxiety over the prospect of informing a pet owner of a poor prognosis than over the prospect of actually losing the pet. While it is impossible to separate the experience of the loss from the need to interact with owners over the loss, the veterinarians interviewed made a clear distinction that owner-clinician interactions heightened stressfulness of the work.

In exploring this issue in depth, veterinarians behaved as though they held themselves responsible for pleasing the anxious pet owner (Wessells 1979). Veterinarians reported feeling anxious if the owner appeared visibly upset either on presenting the pet, or on leaving after treatment was rendered. This observation of the owners resulted in the veterinarians' feeling they needed to do something. Hence their behavior became motivated by what they felt would please the owner.

The consequence of holding oneself responsible for pleasing pet owners was to condition veterinarians to expect to be able to cure the pet. The effects of this expectation on the owner-clinician interaction were many. When veterinarians were faced with an anxious pet owner, they moved in a natural direction; they focused on the pet's ailments. This pattern resulted in the veterinarians' overlooking the anxiety in the owner. The consequence of this pattern can be best seen in the following hypothetical case.

An anxious-looking pet owner presents an injured pet. The owner is minimally communicative. The clinician, sensing the tension, begins vigorously questioning the owner concerning the history of the injury. The owner becomes more anxious and less communicative. At this point the clinician becomes frustrated, and so the pattern spirals.

What becomes obvious is that the clinician's expectation of pleasing the pet owner by curing the pet led to increased tension in the pet owner–veterinarian dyad. This increase in tension further frustrated the course of treatment and increased the stressfulness of the encounter.

Observing such a situation raises questions concerning what would be helpful to veterinarians in coping with these types of situations. Like psychotherapists, veterinarians can begin by developing a definition of their responsibilities to the pet and family that is based on what they can realistically do, not on the outcome of their efforts. Veterinarians cannot be responsible for all the factors that influence the recuperation of a pet. Nor can veterinarians be responsible for pleasing the pet owner. Should veterinarians assume these responsibilities they would be imposing unrealistic expectations on themselves. Veterinarians can be responsible for providing quality services. To define responsibility in this manner would serve to disengage veterinary success from pet cure, thus enabling veterinarians to set more realistic goals based on their own professional behavior.

This is only a starting point in learning to cope with these stressful situations, since intellectual definitions of one's responsibility are usually forgotten in the face of an anxiety-provoking situation. What such an effort does afford the veterinarian is a benchmark with which to monitor her or his ability to follow through with intellectually defined behavior that may feel inappropriate at times of high anxiety generated from encounters with anxious pet owners (Price and Bergen 1977). It is important to keep in mind that if the veterinarian does manage to operate according to what s/he has intellectually defined as appropriate, the behavior may feel inappropriate. If the clinician is able to persist in this behavior, the dissonance between what s/he does and how s/he feels about what s/he does will eventually subside (Maltsby 1975). The importance of this effort is that it enables veterinarians to define success in terms of their own behavior as opposed to changes in others, whether they are pets or humans. This enables veterinarians to experience more rewards from their careers.

Second, it is important for veterinarians to fully appreciate the appropriateness of owner upset over a pet medical emergency. Numerous studies in the psychiatric literature depict pets in today's society as filling the role of surrogate relatives (Keddie 1977; Levinson 1978; Rynearson 1978). In elevating pets in this way, they come to serve as substitutes for human relationships. Such substitutions run the course from replacing extended family members in a nuclear family society to serving as a sibling to an only child, to replacing the loss of a human relationship with a pet relationship. In some extreme cases, pets have become so important that owners experienced a pathological grief reaction when the pet died, resulting in a brief psychiatric hospitalization for the owners. One of the few empirical studies on the role of pets in the human family found pets humanized by being given human names, the acquisition of pets to replace a loss from human relationships, and also that 8 percent of the respondents felt closer to the family pet than to any human family member (Caine 1979). This study and others support the notion that family dynamics and communication patterns change noticeably with the acquisition of a pet as the following quotation illustrates (Levinson 1978, 1033):

When a pet is introduced into a family, the entire climate of family interaction changes and becomes more complex. Not only does each member of the family interact with the animal in his own characteristic way, but family members interact with each other over the pet. Feelings of rivalry, possessiveness, jealousy can emerge just as with the advent of a new child or sibling.

The role and importance of pets in the family can best be understood through the use of a concept developed by Murray Bowen, M.D., called the emotional triangle. Bowen states that if anxiety increases in a two person relationship, it is predictable for the twosome to focus on a third person, object, or idea. By such a focus the twosome is afforded a sense of closeness while at the same time avoiding anxiety-provoking issues in their two party relationship. This process operates much in the way that scape-goating works (people can gain a sense of closeness at the expense of a common enemy). Bowen and others have written at length on a particular form of emotional triangle that is referred to as the child-focus triangle (Barragan 1976; Bowen 1978; Bradt and Moynihan 1972). In this triangle the parents' main or only source of disagreement is how to handle the child. Issues in the marriage, such as dominance of one spouse over another, control, or conflict expression get channeled around child issues. This results in spouses' taking positions polarized from each other concerning what is best for the child. The child-focused triangle ensures that the child gets inconsistent messages concerning what is appropriate, thus covertly reinforcing inappropriate behavior, often exacerbating normal developmental difficulties. The couple's fights over child issues serve to mask the true conflict. While this is far from a satisfactory adjustment in the family, the parents' focus on the child's real or perceived problems supports a balance or homeostasis in the family emotional process. In such families, if the child's symptoms grew remarkably better or worse, the stability of the family would be threatened since a change in either direction might rob the couple of a source of triangular focus. Hence changes in the child's symptoms produce a significant emotional impact on the family's emotional stability.

Pets are triangled into a family relationship system in much the same way as the symptomatic child (Caine 1979; Entin 1981; Keddie 1977; Levinson 1978; Rynearson 1978; Wessells 1979). Serious medical issues affecting the pet have the potential for radically affecting the family's emotional stability by forcing the family to face the possibility of a loss of the object of their triangular focus. Obviously the intensity of this impact is related to how much the family needs the emotional triangle for family stability. However, even in healthy families where the triangular process is mild, pet loss causes a reshuffling of relationships.

While it is not the goal of my work to train veterinarians as family therapists, it seems important to adequately impart the concept of emotional triangles as a means of understanding and appreciating owner anxiety as well as learning to cope effectively with it.

An illustration may prove helpful at this point. A case was reported to me in which a man came to an emergency animal clinic late at night with an injured pet. The man seemed clearly annoyed, asked questions about costs, and was an all-around nuisance. The clinicians were able to use the concept of triangles to comprehend what superficially appeared to be bizarre owner behavior (people who care enough about their pet to seek emergency treatment typically do not act this way). They decided that the pet was quite close to the man's wife. She was probably too upset to bring in the pet. The man's resentment stemmed mostly from his jealousy of his wife's closeness with the pet coupled by his own inability to choose not to carry the pet for treatment in the face of her upset. The only outlet the owner had for his resentment was at the veterinary clinic. Using the concept of triangles enabled the veterinarian to make sense out of behavior that on the surface appeared bizarre. The man's angry attitude in the veterinary clinic was unexpressed anger at his wife, which became expressed around the pet injury. With this as a working premise, the veterinarian had some idea of how to approach the pet owner.

Using this view of emotional triangles that involve a pet, it is reasonable to look on a pet crisis as a crisis for the family. With this view the veterinarian can expand the unit of treatment from the pet to the pet and the owners. Since in the veterinary profession more than in most others family involvement is crucial (to obtain needed history, for example), it is necessary to develop techniques for dealing with anxious pet owners.

The model from which I draw these techniques is based on the Bowen Theory, a model of family systems psychotherapy (Bowen 1978). As in all psychotherapies, Bowen Theory focuses in part on how people communicate—the elements of communication being the subject of discussion and the feelings associated with it. Relating to someone during anxiety-provoking events requires some degree of focus on feelings as well as content. Failure to do so results in such encounters as that involving the noncommunicative pet owner. In such instances, the owner's attention is usually dominated more by her or his feeling system than thinking system. It becomes necessary to recognize this in the interviewee process to allow owners time to talk about their feelings. This will enable them to begin to talk meaningfully about the pet problem.

Bowen Theory offers techniques that afford the clinician the ability to monitor the dynamic interaction of content and feelings during the course of an interview. The Bowen model is designed with two goals in mind. One is to lower anxiety in the interviewees. The second is to have each person articulate her or his position in relation to the situation. The latter refers to having each interviewee define her or his position in the primary emotional triangle in the family so that s/he can develop means of dealing with the triangling process. Obviously the second goal is of less importance here since the goal of the veterinary interview is to learn about the pet problem, not realign family dynamics. However, it may be helpful to understand some of the second goal in order to learn how to intervene with the family. For example, if we use the case of the angry pet owner coming to the clinic, we find it may be necessary to learn enough about his point in the family triangle to understand and appreciate the feeling part of his communication.

The Bowenian model of intervention is helpful in accomplishing the goals of calming the family and identifying the owners' parts in the emotional triangle and facilitating pet treatment in a number of ways. First, communication with the pet owners is channeled through the clinician. This enables the clinician to structure the process of the interview. While it is often necessary to have pet owners talk about feelings to reduce anxiety and facilitate information gathering regarding the pet problem, it is necessary for the veterinarian to limit the amount of feeling-oriented dialogue. To permit owners to talk overly long about their feelings, may delay treatment to the animal and demand too much of the clinician's time. For these reasons, the veterinarian needs to have a leadership role in the interview. The clinician's role then is to keep the discussion going and focused, but to refrain from trying to influence people's comments. Pet owners talking with each other about the pet problem reinforces their anxiety. For that reason, the veterinarian is most effective using a Bowenian interview format that directs questions to each owner. There are several advantages to using a questioning format. First, the veterinarian's use of questions encourages the pet owners to defer to the clinician to structure the interview process. Second, the alert veterinarian can direct questions so as to gather information or explore owner feelings, thus shifting the focus from information to owner anxiety much more quickly than does use of a declarative style interview format. By limiting the focus of questions to *when, where, who, what,* and *how* (not *why*), the pet owners are encouraged to stay with their thinking system rather than move into their feeling system. The use of *why* questions is detrimental to the interview process since it encourages pet owners to be more aware of their feelings, not actions. Thus anxiety is heightened. With each pet owner the clinician needs to find the necessary balance that adequately addresses both information gathering and the owner's anxiety so that the pet owner can report adequately on the pet problem. If owners begin to manifest their anxiety to the detriment of giving information about the pet, focus needs to be temporarily redirected to the owners' anxiety. The clinician can manage these shifts from objectivity to owner anxiety, as noted earlier, by asking questions directed at either the owner's thinking or feeling. Hence the use of a Bowenian model of intervention accomplishes the goals of calming the family, understanding the triangular process, and facilitating pet treatment.

It is important for the clinician to keep in mind that the manifestation of upset in an owner is appropriate and understandable when viewed within the context of the owner's relationship system, her or his family, both human and pet. The clinician cannot be responsible for changing these feelings, only attempting to understand them and work with them in the manner described above so that the pet treatment can be facilitated.

As a family therapist, I am interested in the impact on the

family of a serious pet injury or pet loss. In this chapter, I have dealt with how pet owner anxiety over a serious pet injury or threatened loss gets carried over to the owner-clinician relationship. Consequently the focus of this presentation has been primarily on the family dynamics in a family experiencing a pet-related crisis and the pet owner–clinician encounter.

Two additional points that were not a direct part of what was covered merit discussion; however, they influence the clinician's tolerance to cope with these encounters. The first involves interpersonal issues among the staff members. The relationship one shares with coworkers can prove either helpful or detrimental in coping with the stresses generated from frequent encounters with families in crisis over their pet. Gaining emotional support and cooperation from coworkers is especially helpful in a stressful work environment. The more staff members are able to resolve interpersonal conflicts, the more they can gain support from each other. Since this is a crucial consideration, I would suggest that veterinary clinicians, as part of their work routine, establish a time when interpersonal issues can be appropriately addressed.

The final point to be stressed is the ability of the clinician to affect the work environment positively. I believe we all have limits concerning how we function in our work roles. I also believe that within those limits we have some degree of latitude to enable us to structure our work more to meet our needs. This could mean anything from rearranging a desk top, to realigning work schedules, to deciding to see anxious clients in a different environment (a more private room) that may serve to calm them down. It is important for people to function in a work role that enhances their self-esteem and brings them gratification. In so doing satisfied workers bring more to their work setting. Therefore it is important for clinicians to be aware of and attend to their own needs before engaging the public.

I have presented a brief overview of the family therapy concepts and ideas that I believe relate favorably to the veterinary setting. I chose a family model since the literature suggests that pet loss, or the concern about pet loss, makes a significant impact on the family emotional system. In turn, families in crisis over a potential pet loss present the veterinarian with a treatment unit that encompasses more than the medical issues involved in the pet emergency.

The connectedness of these relationships is perhaps best summed up in a quotation by Chief Sealth of the Duwanish Tribe, State of Washington, in a letter to the President of the United States, 1855:

What is man without beast? If all the beasts were gone, men would die from great loneliness of spirit, for whatever happens to the beast also happens to man. All things are connected. Whatever befalls the earth befalls the sons of the earth.

REFERENCES

Barragan, M. 1976. The child-centered family. In *Family therapy: Theory and practice,* ed. P. J. Guerin, Jr. New York: Gardner.
Bowen, M. 1978. *Family therapy in clinical practice.* New York: Aaronson.
Bradt, J., and C. Moynihan. 1972. Opening the safe: A study of child-focused families. In *Systems therapy,* ed. J. O. Bradt, and C. J. Moynihan. Washington, D.C.: Bradt and Moynihan.
Caine, A. 1979. A study of pets in the family system. In *Georgetown symposia,* vol. IV, ed. R. Sager. Washington, D.C.: Ruth Sager.
Entin, A. 1981. Family icons: Photographs in family psychotherapy. In *The newer therapies: A workbreak,* ed. L. Abt, and I. Stuart. New York: Van Nostrand.
Keddie, K. 1977. Pathological mourning after the death of a domestic pet. *British Journal of Psychiatry* 131:21–25.
Larson, C., D. Gilbertson, and J. Powell. 1978. Therapist burnout: Perspectives on a critical issue. *Social Casework* 59:563–65.
Levinson, B. 1978. Pets and personality development. *Psychological Reports* 42:1031–38.
Maltsby, M. 1975. *Help yourself to happiness through rational self-counseling.* Boston: Herman Publishing.
Price, T., and B. Bergen. 1977. The relationship to death as a source of stress for nurses on a coronary care unit. *Omega* 8:229–38.
Rynearson, E. K. 1978. Humans and pets and attachment. *British Journal of Psychiatry* 133:550–55.
Wessells, D. T. 1979. *Systems-based psychological education program for stress reduction in emergency veterinary personnel: Development and evaluation.* Advanced Certificate Project Working Paper I. College of William and Mary, unpublished manuscript.

22

Epilogue:
A Historical Perspective

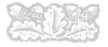

E G I L D E   S E R A V A L L I

SINCE PREHISTORIC TIMES humans have had pets as companions. It is thought that the first pet was the dog, who became a helper in hunting. And it is known that Egyptians, attributing divinity to cats, kept them in their houses and temples. However, the recorded history of the relationships of pets with humans comes largely from the Greeks and the Romans. In ancient Greece birds were frequently kept as pets. Drawings on Greek pottery and sculptures, showing humans with birdlike characteristics and birds with human characteristics, suggest that the Greeks recognized resemblances between the two species. Whether they ever regarded birds as gods or invested animals with a sense of the divine is still doubtful, even if images of these creatures have been used to represent the souls of the dead.

The Greeks' attachment for their pets was so intense they expressed sorrow at a pet's death by writing an epitaph. When a pet partridge was killed by the household cat, the bird's owner wrote (Pollard 1977, 138):

No more, poor partridge, exiled from the rocks does your wicker cage contain you, nor with the brilliance of the bright-eyed down do you rustle the tips of your sun-warmed feathers. The cat bit your head off, but I seized all the rest, and did not satisfy her savage jaws. Now shall the dust not lie light on you, but heavy, lest she drug out your remains.

Later, the same poet turns against the miscreant in stronger terms (p. 138:)

Does the house-cat expect to go on living in my house after eating my partridge? No, I will not permit, dear partridge, your passing to go unavenged, for on your course I will slay your foe.

Inspired by the accident, a friend of the owner also wrote an epigram expressing his anger at the cat (p. 138):

Cat, you wretch, rival of man-killing hounds, you are one of Acteon's fell monsters. By eating this partridge you have brought sorrow to your master, just as if you had eaten him yourself. You have now set your mind on partridges. Meantime, the mice play, making off with your scraps.

In the *Odyssey*, Homer describes the death of Argos, the old and sick loyal dog of Odysseus. He could finally die in peace and with grace after his master has returned and he has recognized him before anyone else.

> While he [Odysseus] spoke
> an old hound, lying near, pricked up his ears
> and lifted up his muzzle. This was Argos,
> trained as a puppy by Odysseus,
> but never taken on a hunt before
> his master sailed for Troy. The young men, afterward,
> hunted wild goats with him, and hare, and deer,
> but he had grown old in his master's absence,
> treated as rubbish now, he lay at last
> upon a mass of dung before the gates —
> manure of mules and cows, piled there until
> fieldhands could spread it on the king's estate.
> Abandoned there, and half destroyed with flies,
> old Argos lay.
>   But when he knew he heard
> Odysseus' voice nearby, he did his best
> to wag his tail, nose down, with flattened ears,
> having no strength to move nearer his master.
> And the man looked away,
> wiping a salt tear from his cheek; but he
> hid this from Eumaios. Then he said:
> "I marvel that they leave this hound to lie
> here on the dung pile;
> he would have been a fine dog, from the look of him,

though I can't say as to his power and speed
when he was young. You find the same good build
in house dogs, table dogs, landowners keep
all for style."
   And you reply, Eumaios:
"A hunter owned him—but the man is dead
in some far place. If this old hound could show
the form he had when lord Odysseus left him,
going to Troy, you'd see him swift and strong.
He never shrank from any savage thing
he'd brought to bay in the deep woods; on the scent
no other dog kept up with him. No misery
has him lash. His owner died abroad,
and here the women slaves will take no care of him . . . ,"
but death and darkness in that instant closed the
eyes of Argos, who had seen his master,
Odysseus, after twenty years.

Argos' behavior brings up questions about animals' perceptions. What is it that allows them to recognize the master? Only
smell? It seems as if Argos was waiting for his master's return
before dying. It was almost as though he "knew" his master would
return home, and he hung on, waiting, not letting himself go. It is
interesting to note that today's approach to death focuses on "let
me go" and "I let you go" between the dying and the survivors.
Here, the subtle link was between an animal and a human.

The Romans, breaking away from the Greek tradition, had
funerals and erected tombs when a pet died. During the reign of
Tiberius (A.D. 36), a raven chick flew down from the temple of
Castor to the nearby shop of a cobbler. The little bird was welcomed by the owner as a religious symbol. The creature soon
learned to talk and flew every morning to the Forum where it
greeted the Emperor. It performed the same feat for several years
and gained great renown. A tenant in a neighboring shop became
envious of the cobbler's success as a result of the remarkable bird.
One day the bird befouled his shoes with its droppings, and the
man killed the animal in a sudden fit of anger. This aroused such a
storm of indignation that the killer of the bird was driven from the
neighborhood and murdered. The dead bird was given a funeral as
though it were a human. An enormous crowd attended the rite,
and the draped bier was carried on the shoulders of two Ethio-
pians. The procession was led by a piper and wreaths were put

around the pyre erected on the Appian Way (Pollard 1977, 136). In those ancient times, even eagles were kept as pets and proved to be most affectionate. King Pirrus had an eagle which was so attached to him that when he died, the bird pined until it died itself.

Birds' affection toward children is also recorded. Pollard writes about two eaglets belonging to a boy and a girl. When the children died at a very young age, as often occurred in those days, the birds flew onto the funeral pyres and burned with their owners.

Today, many similar stories are heard or read, indicating that the relationship between humans and animals seems to be universal and unchangeable. Since this kind of relationship is based on reciprocal love, the expression of this basic feeling between human and animal must change according to modern custom. Where once animals cast themselves into the flames of the funeral pyre, we now read of animals dying of starvation and grief near the graves of their owners.

Animals' knowledge of or instinct about death has been questioned. Some facts indicate that animals are aware that life has to come to an end. For instance, they often appear to have a presentiment of approaching death and lie down in anticipation of it; they show sadness and signs of mourning when their companion or their puppy dies; they also simulate death in order to escape danger and to deceive a potential enemy.

Other interpretations of animal instincts about death deny that they have such knowledge. When animals lie down before dying, it is explained, the cause is simply weakness induced by old age or sickness. However, each species of animal seems to behave in a specific and unique way. Rats remove the body of the dead member of the community and avoid eating the food that might have caused the death. Among monkeys, the dead are kept in the community and offered food, as if they were still alive.

Another controversial question concerns whether animals know when they are dying. To a certain extent we can say yes. Sick or severely wounded cats, dogs, horses, and birds, lie down in an apparent state of resignation and reject any food. It has been suggested that it is the species, not the individual, that knows death. Since death means loss of the individual but not of the species, it is necessary to understand the relationship between the individual and the species in order to speculate on animals' awareness of death.

Historically, then, it appears that the person who feels the need of an uncritical companion has always looked to animals. And all evidence shows animals need to be loved and appreciated for what they give. These inner qualities are expressed in different ways and with characteristics common among all living creatures, especially the wish to give one's best for the benefit of those whom one loves.

REFERENCE

Pollard, J. 1977. *Birds in Greek life and myth.* Plymouth, England: Thames and Hudson.

CONTRIBUTORS

EDITORS

WILLIAM J. KAY, D.V.M., chief of staff, Animal Medical Center, New York

HERBERT A. NIEBURG, PH.D., professor of Community Health, Long Island University (Westchester Division); attending psychotherapist, Animal Medical Center, New York

AUSTIN H. KUTSCHER, D.D.S., president, The Foundation of Thanatology; professor of Dentistry (in psychiatry), Department of Psychiatry, College of Physicians and Surgeons, Columbia University, New York

ROSS M. GREY, D.V.M., professor of Comparative Pathology; chairman, Institute of Comparative Medicine, College of Physicians and Surgeons, Columbia University, New York

CAROLE E. FUDIN, PH.D., C.S.W., A.S.C.W., attending psychotherapist, Animal Medical Center; private practice, New York

LILLIAN G. KUTSCHER, publications editor, The Foundation of Thanatology, New York

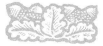

JACOB ANTELYES, D.V.M., private practice, Middle Village, N.Y.

ALAN M. BECK, SC.D., director, Center for Interaction of Animals and Society, School of Veterinary Medicine, University of Pennsylvania, Philadelphia

ESTHER BRAUN, M.S.W., social worker, Pediatric Service, The Presbyterian Hospital in the City of New York

LEO K. BUSTAD, D.V.M., PH.D., dean, College of Veterinary Medicine, Washington State University, Pullman

M. W. FOX, D.SC., B.VET. Med., PH.D., director, Institute for the Study of Animal Problems, Washington, D.C.

ERIKA FRIEDMANN, PH.D., assistant professor of Health Sciences, Brooklyn College of the City University of New York, Brooklyn; lecturer in Animal Ecology, School of Veterinary Medicine, University of Pennsylvania, Philadelphia

PATRICK HAFNER, D.V.M., Boulevard Animal Clinic, East Lansing, Mich.

JAMES M. HARRIS, D.V.M., Montclair Veterinary Clinic and Hospital, Oakland, Calif.

LINDA M. HINES, M.A., College of Veterinary Medicine, Washington State University, Pullman

AARON A. KATCHER, M.D., associate professor of Psychiatry, University of Pennsylvania, Philadelphia

BORIS M. LEVINSON, PH.D., psychotherapist, Blueberry Treatment Centers, Inc., Brooklyn, N.Y.; emeritus professor of Psychology, Yeshiva University, New York

MARY LINK, therapeutic riding instructor, Green Chimneys Farm, Brewster, N.Y.

JAMES J. LYNCH, PH.D., professor of Psychiatry, School of Medicine, University of Maryland, Baltimore

MICHAEL J. McCULLOCH, M.D., Northwest Psychiatric Associates, Portland, Oreg.

GEORGE PAULUS, PH.D., Michigan State University, East Lansing

JAMIE QUACKENBUSH, M.S.W., A.C.S.W., instructor, School of Veterinary Medicine, University of Pennsylvania, Philadelphia

BERNARD E. ROLLIN, PHD., professor of Philosophy, Colorado State University, Fort Collins

MARC A. ROSENBERG, V.M.D., adjunct associate in Medicine, School of Veterinary Medicine, University of Pennsylvania, Philadelphia; Co-Director, Cherry Hill Animal Hospital, Cherry Hill, N.J.

ELEANOR L. RYDER, M.A., M.S.W., associate professor of Social Work, School of Social Work, University of Pennsylvania, Philadelphia

E. K. RYNEARSON, M.D., Department of Medicine, Section of Psychiatry, The Mason Clinic, Seattle

EGILDE SERAVALLI, PH.D., research associate, Department of Anesthesiology, Beth Israel Hospital and Medical Center, New York

CYRUS S. STEWART, PH.D., Michigan State University, East Lansing

WILLIAM H. SULLIVAN, D.V.M., director, The Cat Practice, New York

SUE A. THOMAS, R.N., PH.D., assistant professor, School of Nursing and Department of Psychiatry and Human Behavior, University of Maryland, Baltimore

JOHN C. THRUSH, M.A., M.P.H., public health consultant, Division of Chronic Disease Control, Department of Public Health, State of Michigan, Lansing

VICTORIA A. VOITH, D.V.M., associate professor of Medicine, School of Veterinary Medicine, University of Pennsylvania, Philadelphia

SALLY OBLAS WALSHAW, M.A., V.M.D., assistant professor, Animal Technology Program, Michigan State University, East Lansing

D. T. WESSELS, JR., ED.D., supervisor of counseling, Alternatives, Inc., Newport News, Va.

All royalties from the sale of this text are assigned to The Foundation of Thanatology, a not-for-profit, tax-exempt, public foundation devoted to scientific and humanistic inquiries as well as to the application of knowledge to the subjects of the psychological aspects of dying; reactions to death, loss and grief; and recovery from bereavement.

INDEX